THE
# Good Health
## DIRECTORY

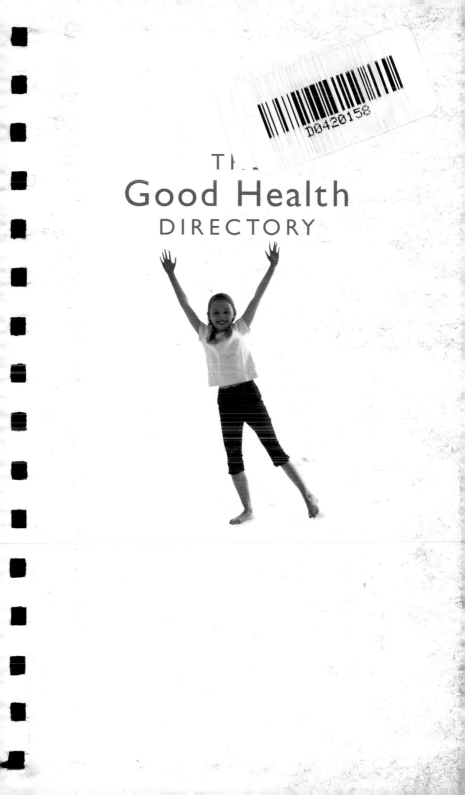

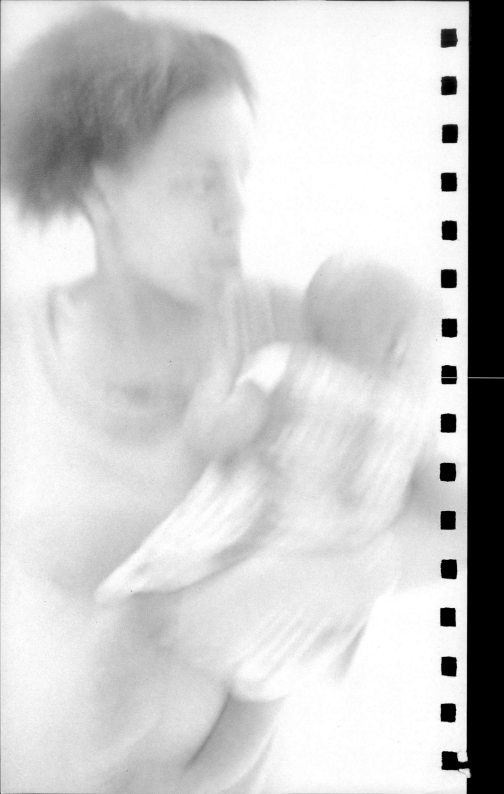

# THE
# Good Health
# DIRECTORY

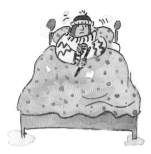

CONSULTANT EDITOR
## MICHAEL VAN STRATEN

FOREWORD BY
## C. NORMAN SHEALY, MD, PhD

CONTRIBUTORS
## NAOMI CRAFT
## JOSIE DRAKE
## FIONA DRY
## PENELOPE ODY
## MICHAEL VAN STRATEN

Newleaf

CONTRIBUTORS
*Main introduction, ailment introductions, Kitchen Medicine,*
*Nutrition, Prevention:* MICHAEL VAN STRATEN
*Aromatherapy:* JOSIE DRAKE
*Conventional Medicine:* NAOMI CRAFT
*Herbal Remedies:* PENELOPE ODY
*Homeopathic Remedies:* FIONA DRY

First published in 2000 by
Newleaf
an imprint of
GILL & MACMILLAN LTD
Goldenbridge, Dublin 8
with associated companies throughout the world
www.gillmacmillan.ie
ISBN 0 7171 2995 0

*Note from the publisher*
Information given in this book is not intended to be
taken as a replacement for medical advice. Any person with
a condition requiring medical attention should consult
a qualified medical practitioner or therapist.

This book was conceived, designed
and produced by
THE IVY PRESS LIMITED
The Old Candlemakers
West Street
Lewes, East Sussex BN7 2NZ

*Creative Director:* PETER BRIDGEWATER
*Designer:* JANE LANAWAY
*DTP Designer:* CHRIS LANAWAY
*Editorial Director:* DENNY HEMMING
*Managing Editor:* ANNE TOWNLEY
*Editor:* MANDY GREENFIELD
*Studio Photography:* MARIE-LOUISE AVERY, WALTER GARDINER,
IAN PARSONS, GUY RYECART
*Illustrations:* MADELEINE HARDIE
*Models:* MARK JAMIESON
*Picture research:* TRUDI VALTER
*US Medical Consultant:* MELISSA STILES, MD,
University of Wisconsin, Madison Department of Family Education

Originated and printed in China by Hong Kong Graphic and Printing Ltd

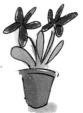

# Contents

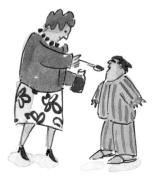

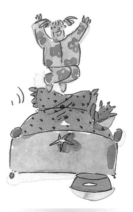

### Caution buttons

*The colour of the circular button at the corner of each caution box indicates the therapy to which that caution relates:*

- **CONVENTIONAL MEDICINE**
- **HOMEOPATHIC REMEDIES**
- **HERBAL REMEDIES**
- **NUTRITION**
- **AROMATHERAPY**
- **GENERAL WARNING**

# Foreword

It has been estimated that well over 90 per cent of the improvement in life expectancy in the Western world is the result of the chlorination of water, adequate sewage disposal, the pasteurization of milk and adequate calorie intake. Now however in the West, and in the United States In particular, we eat too many calories, and that fact alone accounts for many of the diseases that cause premature death. Dr John Knowles, late President of the Rockefeller Foundation, estimated that 85 per cent of illnesses are actually the result of poor lifestyle choices.

In addition to choosing *good health* habits to preserve your health and quality of life, only a limited number of illnesses actually require medical attention. At least 80 per cent of all illnesses are best treated in 'the folk domain', with the time-honoured, safe approaches detailed in this beautifully illustrated book. Immediate medical attention is essential when there is sudden severe pain in the head, chest or abdomen; paralysis or numbness; loss of consciousness; seizures; fever above 39.5°C/103°F; difficulty in breathing; confusion or significant personality changes; an irregular or very rapid heartbeat or a sudden drop in heart rate below 50 beats per minute; significant swelling or redness of any part of the body; inability to urinate or defecate; significant bleeding; rapid weight loss, especially in conjunction with frequent urination and excessive thirst; a sore that does not heal; change in a wart or mole; frequent indigestion or trouble swallowing; a significant change in bowel habits; a persistent cough or hoarseness; a lump in the breast or scrotum – these problems represent the 15 per cent of illnesses that are best treated with modern medicine.

For the vast majority of symptoms, however, which are signs of stress that has not yet produced worrisome illness, self-responsibility is well advised. *The Good Health Directory* provides the superb answers you need in order to be well informed and responsible.

C. NORMAN SHEALY, MD, PhD

# Introduction

There is nothing new about home remedies. Since the time of man's most primitive homes – in caves and mud huts, the tree-houses of the tropical rainforest and the igloos of the frozen wastes, the crofter's cottage and the Native North American wigwam, the monastery and the medieval castle – people have used home remedies in order to treat their everyday ailments and promote good health.

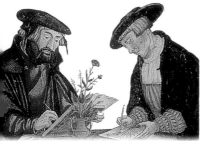

**ABOVE** Herbalism has been used as a healing therapy for centuries.

Such remedies have been passed down from generation to generation – in the Western world, usually from mother to daughter – and, until quite recently, featured strongly in every cookery book, in which there was always a section on food suitable for the sickroom.

This book collects together the ancient wisdom of herbal medicine, the more modern applications of homeopathy, the expertise of conventional medicine, the gentle effectiveness of aromatherapy and age-old nutritional practice, together with a few basic exercises. (For some entries at the end of each system we have included the most immediately beneficial therapies.) It tells you not only how to deal with minor health problems, but how to utilize home remedies to relieve some of the discomforts of complex diseases.

From homeopathic pillules for sinusitis to horse-chestnut ointment for varicose veins, from pumpkin seeds and brazil nuts to combat infection to the **BRAT** diet for diarrhoea, from lavender oil for insomnia to dandelions for cystitis, there are answers for dozens of everyday health problems contained within this book. What is more, these are gentle answers, to which more and more people are turning in order to avoid unnecessary medication with powerful drugs – many of which are now available over the counter – and endless prescriptions for sleeping pills, tranquillizers and painkillers, as well as antibiotics.

Many 'alternative practitioners' talk about the good old days before we had a pharmaceutical industry, but this is simply living in cloud-cuckoo-land. All treatments and medicines must be viewed in the light of risk and benefit, and it is doubtless true that most natural therapies represent minimal risk and valuable benefit. But the advances of modern medicine and surgery, plus the life-saving benefits of sophisticated pharmaceuticals, cannot be dismissed.

Though many of the remedies in this book are an alternative to other treatments, there is really no such thing as 'alternative medicine' – only good and bad medicine. In serious illness the patient is best served by a combination of the most suitable therapies for their particular problem, and this is why the term 'complementary medicine' is used. When doctors and other practitioners work together, the patient reaps the greatest benefit.

This book is not meant as a substitute for your doctor, though in many instances the safe, simple treatments suggested will help prevent unnecessary trips to the surgery. Remember, though, that first aid is just what it says, and if you are in any doubt as to the seriousness of a symptom – especially when it involves children – then see your doctor. Most parents have a natural instinct about the health of their children, and if your gut instinct is worrying you, then do not delay in seeking medical help.

Most accidents occur in the home – more than half of us have an accident each year that requires some sort of treatment, and one-fifth of us suffer an injury that requires us to undergo medical treatment of one kind or another.

**BELOW** Children, too, can benefit from treatment with complementary medicines.

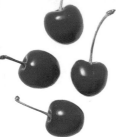

**ABOVE** Cherries contain vitamin C and bioflavonoids.

Common sense and care can help to make accidents less likely, but it takes a bit more effort to prevent many of the other ailments described in this book. However, making the effort is well worth while and you will find detailed advice on how improving your nutrition can help you avoid recurring problems; how aromatherapy can soothe and de-stress you; and how, using the other home remedies, you can boost your resistance to everyday infections.

In today's over-complicated, technological and stressful world many of us are anxious to take more control of our own lives. Using the home remedies in this book is one step in that direction, and we hope that the information we have provided will give you the self-confidence and the knowledge that you need to tackle many common ailments. Most of the remedies have stood the test of time and can now claim scientific validation. Others are included on the basis of centuries of use and a vast body of anecdotal evidence. Although scientists may scoff, modern medicine has been built on the observations and anecdotes of great practitioners of the healing arts, and some of the most powerful modern drugs were in common use long before clinical trials were even invented.

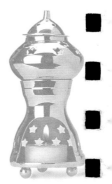

**ABOVE** A simple vaporizer for burning oils.

We hope that you will quickly discover the many benefits of these simple remedies and, by passing them on to your relatives and friends, will add to the vast body of anecdotal evidence and old wives' tales that really help in promoting natural good health.

**MICHAEL VAN STRATEN**

# The Immune System

Over the last 20 years or so an inefficient immune system has become the catch-all culprit for every day-to-day health problem. Yet few people are aware of the extent to which a healthy lifestyle can strengthen their immune systems, and of the importance of this body system in repelling those 'ordinary' illnesses that beset all of us at times. This section looks at the health problems – fever, flu, sore throat, and so on – that can arise from a poorly functioning immune system, and at the best treatments for them, drawn from a variety of disciplines.

# Infections: bacterial/viral

*Characterized by a fever; other symptoms depend on the underlying cause, but may include muscular aches and pains; shivering; localized soreness and inflammation; sore throat and blocked sinuses.*

**W**e share the world we live in with teeming billions of bacteria and viruses. Many have no impact on the human species, some cause minor discomfort, while others cause life-threatening disease. Our natural defence system is a delicate mechanism that needs careful nurturing, and when we ignore its needs we can expect to reap a bitter harvest of ill health, disability and even death. Nurturing this system starts and finishes in the home.

## Call the doctor

*If very high temperatures, above 39°C (102.2°F), do not respond to conventional medication.*

### CONVENTIONAL MEDICINE

When you feel shivery due to a fever, curling up in bed wearing extra clothes may simply make the problem worse. Instead, try a warm bath, which will help restore normal body temperature, or sponging the body with tepid water. Dress in cool clothing and take a pain reliever. Antibiotics may be prescribed, although viruses will not respond to them.

**DOSAGE: ADULTS** 1–2 tablets of pain relievers at onset of fever, repeated every 4 hours; consult pack for details.

**DOSAGE: CHILDREN** Give regular doses of liquid pain reliever; consult pack, or follow medical advice.

### HERBAL REMEDIES

Modern research has shown that many herbs can combat viruses or bacteria.

**USE AND DOSAGE** Echinacea is one of the most effective herbs – take up to 600mg in tablets three times daily at the first sign of infection.

Garlic is both antiviral and antibacterial, so take up to 2g daily in capsules or add 1–2 cloves to cooked dishes.

Chinese tonic herbs, like astragalus, reishi and shi-itake mushrooms will boost the immune system. Try the mushrooms in soups, or buy them in capsules.

## NUTRITION

Building a sound immune system starts three months before conception, with healthy eating by both prospective parents and avoidance of alcohol, large amounts of caffeine, nicotine and drugs. Optimum nutrition means: a minimum of 5 portions a day of fruit and vegetables; lots of complex carbohydrates such as wholemeal bread, brown rice, pasta, cereals and beans; a sensible intake of low-fat dairy products; half a dozen eggs and at least four portions of oily fish each week; and plenty of other fish, poultry and a little red meat.

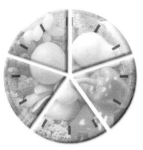

**ABOVE** Eating 5 portions of fruit and vegetables each day is the basis of a healthy diet.

Good nutrition is important throughout life, but at times of particular stress it is absolutely vital. Get your essential minerals by eating a handful of pumpkin seeds every day for their zinc and five brazil nuts daily for their selenium. Vitamins A, C and the all-important E provide a protective antioxidant force, while the high natural bacteria content of live yoghurt is one of the great immune-boosters.

## AROMATHERAPY

- Tea tree *(Melaleuca alternifolia)*
- Lavender *(Lavandula angustifolia)*
- Eucalyptus *(Eucalyptus radiata)*
- Thyme *(Thymus vulgaris)*
- Niaouli *(Melaleuca viridiflora)*
- Bergamot *(Citrus bergamia)*

These oils attack the organisms, kill airborne germs and strengthen the body's immune system.

**APPLICATION** Depends on what is most convenient or pleasant for the user.

> **Caution**
> Always read pain-reliever packages carefully, and do not exceed the stated dose.

## HOMEOPATHIC REMEDIES

In homeopathy the patient is treated according to symptoms that the body produces, and not necessarily according to the type of infection that leads to those symptoms (so look at *Fever* on p.16, *Influenza* on p.18, *Sore Throat* on p.20, etc.).

THYME

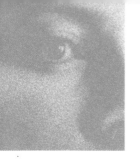

# Allergies

*Characterized by itching skin and/or eyes, sneezing fits and a blocked or runny nose; more severe symptoms may include wheezy breathing, difficulty in swallowing and swollen lips and tongue.*

**BELOW** Wearing a medical allergy necklace can save your life.

**A**n allergy is an abnormal response by the body's natural defence mechanisms, very often to something that would not normally be a hazard. The body wrongly identifies a food, a pollen or an atmospheric pollutant as a dangerous invader; the white cells over-react; and this 'allergic response' then becomes an illness in itself. Sometimes avoidance of the allergen is the only cure; but home remedies can make an enormous difference.

**LEFT** Steroid nasal sprays can bring some relief from allergies for both adults and children.

### ✚ CONVENTIONAL MEDICINE

Mild symptoms can be treated with antihistamines or steroid nose drops. For more severe and potentially fatal allergic reactions, such as some cases of peanut allergy, seek urgent medical attention. If you know you have a severe allergic reaction, wear a MedicAlert bracelet or necklace describing your allergy in case you fall ill.

**DOSAGE: ADULTS** Antihistamines are available as tablets, syrup or eyedrops; some preparations can cause drowsiness. Most tablets are taken once a day; eyedrops more frequently – consult pack for details or follow medical advice. Apply 2 puffs of steroid nose spray per nostril twice a day.

**DOSAGE: CHILDREN** Doses of antihistamine syrup depend on the age of the child; consult pack, or follow medical advice. Apply 2 puffs of steroid nose spray per nostril twice a day to children over six.

### ✿ HOMEOPATHIC REMEDIES

**⚘ Apis 30c**

For swelling around eyes, sometimes too great to open lids. Swollen face, lips and tongue.

**DOSAGE** 1 tablet every 15 minutes. Maximum six doses.

**Caution**

*Violent allergic reactions – anaphylaxis – can be fatal. Sufferers should carry an emergency injection of adrenalin. Breathing difficulties or swelling of the face constitute dire emergencies.*

## NUTRITION

Foods are among the commonest causes of allergic reactions, either through eating them or through contact (see Dermatitis on p.132). Allergies often run in families, but there is evidence that exposure to some foods too early in life (such as cow's milk or peanuts) can also cause problems. The most common food allergens are milk, eggs, dairy products, shellfish, nuts and berries. But allergies – which are very rapid reactions to minute amounts of the culprit – should not be confused with food intolerance, which produces symptoms hours after consumption. Milk intolerance is a very common problem, whereas true milk allergy is quite rare.

All foods that are rich in B vitamins can help reduce the severity of allergic symptoms, and oily fish can help in treating eczema, due to its high content of omega-3 fatty acids.

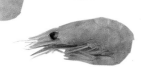

**ABOVE** Some people experience a quick and violent reaction to shrimps and other shellfish.

## HERBAL REMEDIES

Garlic is traditionally used to combat food allergies – add cloves to cooking or take garlic capsules daily. Regular cups of agrimony tea can improve the digestive system's ability to cope with allergens, while marigold will help combat the fungal infections often associated with food allergy. Teas made from camomile, elder or yarrow flowers can also reduce allergic reactions.

GARLIC CAPSULES

> **Caution**
> Several herbs, particularly fresh rue, can trigger allergic reactions. If using true melissa, which is very rare and expensive, be very careful about how you use it, for it can cause nasty burns to the skin.

**BELOW** Marigold is useful for fighting the fungal infections that occur with food allergies.

## AROMATHERAPY

- Melissa (Melissa officinalis)
- Roman camomile (Chamaemelum nobile)
- Lavender (Lavandula angustifolia)

These oils soothe and relax the body after its over-reaction to the external stimulus. They are also calming to the emotions.

**APPLICATION** This will depend on the form that the allergy takes. If there is irritation on the skin, use a compress, soothing baths or a lotion containing a few drops of the oils, rubbed in regularly. If the skin is too irritated to be touched, use a spray.

# Fever

*Classic fever symptoms include shivering and a hot, dry skin as the body temperature rises; there may also be aching limbs and copious perspiration, accompanied by a considerable thirst.*

**A** **fever or high temperature is the body's way of reacting to an attack by invading bacteria or viruses. The body's temperature is strictly regulated and is normally between 36.9° and 37.5°C (98.4° and 99.5°F). As little as half-a-degree change in temperature may make you feel unwell and suggests there is an infection somewhere in the body. In most cases this is self-limiting, and the normal sort of high temperature – as a result of flu, for example – may be left to run its course. However, any prolonged bout of fever for which there is no obvious cause, or very high temperature, must be thoroughly investigated.**

### 🌐 Call the doctor

*If very high temperatures, above 39°C (102.2°F), do not respond to conventional medication; are accompanied by cystitis, headache or abdominal pain; or persist for more than 24 hours.*

### ✚ CONVENTIONAL MEDICINE

Curling up under a duvet when you feel shivery and unwell can raise the body temperature and simply make the problem worse. Instead, try a warm bath, or sponging the body with tepid water. Dress in cool clothing and take a pain reliever. Sometimes antibiotics will be prescribed to treat the cause of the fever.

**DOSAGE: ADULTS** 1–2 tablets of pain relievers at onset of fever, repeated every 4 hours; consult pack for details.

**DOSAGE: CHILDREN** Give regular doses of liquid pain reliever; consult pack for details, or follow medical advice.

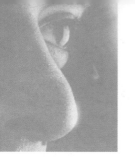

### 🍎 NUTRITION

'Feed a cold and starve a fever' – the old adage is absolutely correct. You will not feel like eating anyway, but the body will lose huge amounts of fluid through sweating, so copious drinks are essential: diluted fresh citrus juices for their immune-boosting vitamin C; pineapple juice for its soothing enzymes (cartons of juice are fine); and herbal teas – camomile, lime blossom and elderflower. Keep your immune system working efficiently by ensuring a regular intake of vitamin C, zinc, selenium and all the carotenoids, by eating a wide variety of fruit and vegetables, nuts and seeds.

**ABOVE** Nuts of all kinds can help to boost the immune system.

## HOMEOPATHIC REMEDIES

**Aconite 30c**

For first stage of illness. Hot, thirsty, anxious and restless. If no improvement move on to:

**Belladonna 30c**

For rapid onset, high fever, red burning face, dry skin, cold feet. Dilated pupils. Hallucinations.

**Gelsemium 30c**

For heavy, aching limbs, reluctance to lift head off pillow. Drowsy, chills up and down spine. No thirst.

DOSAGE 1 tablet every 30 minutes, for six doses, then every 4 hours. Maximum 3 days.

## AROMATHERAPY

**Roman camomile** *(Chamaemelum nobile)*

**Lavender** *(Lavandula angustifolia)*

**Tea tree** *(Melaleuca alternifolia)*

**Juniper** *(Juniperus communis)*

**Peppermint** *(Mentha x piperita)*

Tea tree and juniper encourage the body to sweat, if it needs to eliminate excess fluid. Lavender and peppermint are especially useful for infants, when there is a high temperature that may induce convulsions. Camomile is soothing.

APPLICATION Use either in a bath or in low doses in cool water, to sponge the body down.

## HERBAL REMEDIES

Herbs have long been used in fever management — cooling the body during the 'hot' stages by encouraging sweating (e.g. with yarrow, lime flowers, boneset) and stimulating the digestion (using bitters such as gentian or wormwood), then alternately heating the system during the 'chill' stage (with stimulants like angelica, cinnamon or ginger).

USE AND DOSAGE Confine home remedies to milder cases, using infusions of these herbs as appropriate.

**Caution**

Be particularly alert for fevers starting after trips abroad, after accidents involving cuts and grazes, contact with animals or recent surgery.

YARROW

# Influenza

*High fever; backache and general muscular aches and pains; tiredness and lack of energy, often accompanied by a loss of appetite, sneezing; sore throat and a dry cough; swollen glands in the neck.*

This is an acute viral infection that recurs throughout the population every year. Approximately every three years flu reaches epidemic proportions, as new strains of virus appear to which the general population has no acquired immunity. So make sure that your kitchen cupboard is always equipped with the necessary home remedies.

LOZENGES

### 🌐 Call the doctor

*If a cough is getting worse and you are finding it difficult to breathe.*

**BELOW** Drink plenty of fluids during a bout of flu, especially when you have no appetite for food.

### ➕ CONVENTIONAL MEDICINE

Influenza is caused by a virus infection and so it will not respond to antibiotics. Shivers and muscular aches can be eased by taking pain relievers, while lozenges and hot drinks can help to soothe a sore throat. Rest in bed and make sure you drink plenty of water. Some strains of influenza can be prevented by an annual vaccination.

**DOSAGE: ADULTS** 1–2 tablets of pain reliever at onset of fever, repeated every 4 hours; consult pack for further details.

**DOSAGE: CHILDREN** Give regular doses of liquid pain reliever; consult pack, or follow medical advice.

### ✿ HOMEOPATHIC REMEDIES

🌿 Gelsemium 30c

For drowsiness and heavy lids. Head heavy. Chills up and down spine. No thirst. Weakness and trembling legs. Muscular soreness.

🌿 Eupatorium perfoliatum 30c

For pain in bones and aching muscles in back and limbs. Thirsty. Throbbing headache. Aches and pains better for sweating.

**DOSAGE** 1 tablet every 4 hours until improved. Maximum 12 doses.

## HERBAL REMEDIES

Herbs can help to relieve some of flu's more unpleasant symptoms, as well as combat the debilitation that often follows an attack.

USE AND DOSAGE  Mix equal amounts of boneset, yarrow, elderflower and peppermint and make an infusion with 2tsp per cup and a pinch of cinnamon.

A compress soaked in lavender tea will ease feverish headaches.

As a post-flu tonic, combine a decoction of elecampane root with an equal amount of an infusion of vervain and St John's wort.

## NUTRITION

The time to worry about nutrition and flu is before you get it. So boost your immune system by following the advice given under Infections (see p.12). If you do catch flu, go to bed and stay there for at least 48 hours. For the first 24 hours, take plenty of fluids (lots of lemon juice, hot water and honey as a general soother for the body, and pineapple juice for its healing enzymes) and eat grapes, berries, citrus fruit and ripe pears only. In the second 24 hours, add cooked vegetables and salad. On the third day, add bread, potatoes, rice and pasta. By the fourth day you can resume your normal diet.

CRANBERRIES

During a bout of flu, take 1g of vitamin C three times a day, 5,000 IU of vitamin A and a high-strength B-complex tablet. After a week, reduce the dose to 1g of vitamin C each day, 1,000 IU of vitamin A and the B-complex tablet; continue for at least 3 weeks.

## AROMATHERAPY

Tea tree (Melaleuca alternifolia)
Tea tree will make you sweat, which should help prevent any worse onset.

APPLICATION  Put 4–6 drops into a warm bath and soak; drink a large glass of water and go to bed. Use steam inhalations and burners to stop cross-infection and for symptomatic treatment.

> **Caution**
> *Flu can be complicated by secondary chest infections and possibly pneumonia. The very young, the elderly and anyone with asthma, chronic bronchitis or other obstructive-airways disease, heart disease, kidney problems, diabetes or undergoing immuno-suppressant therapy should get medical help at once.*

**BELOW** Grapes and citrus fruits should be eaten during the early stages of a flu attack.

# Sore throat

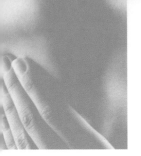

*Characterized by a hoarse, sore voice, which may disappear altogether; or a sore cough; it may follow a cold, overusing the voice or breathing in smoke; sometimes linked to tonsillitis (see p.158).*

**A** sore throat (pharyngitis) may be caused by a viral infection, dehydration, overuse of the voice or shouting (laryngitis), or it may be an early symptom of other infectious diseases. It can also be caused by infection, inflammation and/or enlargement of the tonsils. Sore throats are common and uncomfortable, but they are usually of little clinical significance.

**ABOVE** A sore throat should not generally last for more than a week or so.

## 🌐 Call the doctor

*If there is any change in the quality of your voice that does not return to normal within a week or two; if you have been hoarse for a period of more than 6 weeks.*

### ✚ CONVENTIONAL MEDICINE

Sore vocal cords need rest, which means no talking. Steam inhalations (see p.196) can help to reduce the swelling around the cords and may be used as often as necessary. Linctus or lozenges may help.

**DOSAGE: ADULTS** 1–2 spoonfuls (5–10ml) of linctus or 1 lozenge every 4–5 hours; consult pack for details or follow medical advice.

**DOSAGE: CHILDREN** 1 spoonful (5ml) of linctus or half a lozenge three times daily; consult pack for details, or follow medical advice.

### ▱ HERBAL REMEDIES

Soothing, astringent and antiseptic herbs for use in gargles include sage, lady's mantle, rosemary, thyme, silverweed, agrimony and echinacea.

**USE AND DOSAGE** Make a strong infusion (2–3tsp per cup), strain well and gargle every 30–60 minutes while symptoms persist. (Use the aerial parts of *Echinacea purpurea*, or a root decoction of any of the three available echinacea species.) Fresh *Aloe vera* sap added to the gargle will also help. Drink a standard infusion (1tsp per cup) of any of the above herbs as well.

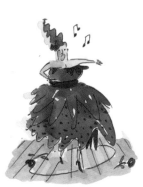

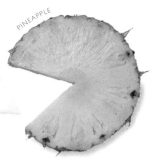

PINEAPPLE

## NUTRITION

For an acute sore throat, especially with a fever, a 24-hour raw fruit and fruit-juice fast will boost the immune system and provide essential nutrients. Drink plenty of pineapple juice and citrus juices diluted 50:50 with water; eat lots of avocados, together with all the exotic fruits, like pineapple, pawpaw and mango. If you are prescribed antibiotics, make sure you have plenty of live yogurt to recondition the natural bugs in your intestines. But the throat's best friend is the kitchen tap: 4–6 glasses of water each day are essential, together with other drinks. And hot water with a dessertspoonful of honey and the juice of half a lemon is one of the most soothing remedies.

## HOMEOPATHIC REMEDIES

🔊 Belladonna 30c

For sudden onset. Throat red, dry, painful, initially on right side. Swallowing very painful.

🔊 Phytolacca 30c

For pain in ears on swallowing. Swallowing hot drinks impossible. Dark red tonsils right side especially swollen. Neck stiff.

🔊 Lachesis 30c

For left-sided pain initially, spreading to right. Sensation of tightness in throat, sensitive to touch. Wakes with sore throat. Difficult to swallow saliva, worse for hot drinks.

DOSAGE 1 tablet every 2 hours for six doses, followed by every 4 hours until improved. Maximum 12 doses.

## AROMATHERAPY

🔊 Sandalwood *(Santalum album)*
🔊 Myrrh *(Commiphora molmol)*
🔊 Tea tree *(Melaleuca alternifolia)*

These oils are antibacterial, fungicidal and help to kill the pain and stop it spreading.

APPLICATION Put the oils into a massage oil or cream and use them on the throat area. Then wrap something warm around the throat.

### Caution

*Recurrent and chronic sore throats may be caused by smoking, excessive alcohol use, repeated vomiting (as in bulimia) or even by a hiatus hernia.*

### Prevention

*To protect your throat, keep your salt consumption to a minimum, drink only modest amounts of alcohol (not spirits), stop smoking and avoid very hot drinks and cola drinks, which irritate the throat's delicate membranes.*

# Shingles

*A burning sensation felt on an area of sensitive skin, which then develops blisters; it most commonly affects an area around the shoulder, chest or waist, or one side of the face and one eye.*

**S**hingles (*Herpes zoster* is its medical name) is caused by the same virus that causes chickenpox. After chickenpox, some of the virus stays dormant in the nerve ganglions for many years. Exposure to chickenpox in later life if you have never had the illness – or to stressful events, physical or emotional – can then catalyse the virus. Up to 20 per cent of adults will be affected, but the elderly and those with a suppressed immune system are at greatest risk. For some, shingles is a mild infection; it leaves others with a wretched condition called 'post-herpetic neuralgia', which may persist for months or even years.

### 🌐 Call the doctor
*If you think you are suffering from shingles.*

**BELOW** Elderly people can be particularly susceptible to shingles.

## ➕ CONVENTIONAL MEDICINE

If you develop symptoms of shingles you may need treatment from your doctor; if the shingles affects your eye, it could cause permanent damage and you should consult your doctor urgently. Antiviral drugs are only effective if given early. Strong pain relievers will also help.

## HERBAL REMEDIES

Shingles responds to a variety of herbal remedies.
USE AND DOSAGE During an attack, echinacea (up to 2g in tablets daily) will help to combat the viral infection.

Drinking plenty of St John's wort infusion may limit the risk of lingering nerve pain, which is so commonly associated with attacks of shingles.

A tea containing equal amounts of passion flower, lemon balm and wild lettuce will also ease the pain and discomfort.

Apply fresh *Aloe vera* sap to any blistering that occurs. Afterwards, use cayenne, vervain or St John's wort in either creams or infused oils in order to combat nerve pain: cayenne is specially effective in this respect.

## AROMATHERAPY

- Eucalyptus *(Eucalyptus radiata)*
- Tea tree *(Melaleuca alternifolia)*
- Lavender *(Lavandula angustifolia)*
- Roman·camomile *(Chamaemelum nobile)*
- Bergamot *(Citrus bergamia)*

These oils are painkilling, antiviral and help to dry out the blisters. Bergamot is active against the *Herpes zoster* virus and is also an antidepressant. Tea-tree oil also helps to build up the body's immune system, so that afterwards the body is more able to fight off infection.

**APPLICATION** Smoothe the oils very gently over the affected area and down either side of the spine, where all the nerve endings are. If the body is too painful to touch, add the oils to a water spray; use a very soft brush to paint the oils on; or use the oils in the bath.

**ABOVE** Eating cherries, eggs and seeds will help to boost your nutrient levels.

## NUTRITION

The B vitamins, bioflavonoids and vitamin C are the key nutrients, so eat plenty of citrus fruit, together with some of the pith and skin between the segments; dark cherries, tomatoes and mangoes; eggs, poultry and liver; nuts, seeds and wholemeal cereals; olive, sunflower and safflower oils. Do not forget that the probiotic bacteria that are present in live yogurt are an essential factor in the body's production of some B vitamins.

## HOMEOPATHIC REMEDIES

- Rhus toxicodendron 6c

For painful, small, watery blisters with a lot of itching. Better for warm applications. Person is restless, which helps to relieve itching. Probably the most common remedy for shingles.

- Ranunculus bulbosus 6c

For burning pain, itching worse for touch. Bluish appearance of spots, which appear in clusters. Neuralgia of the chest wall.

**DOSAGE** 1 tablet every 4 hours until blisters have settled. Maximum 5 days.

### Prevention

*Improved nutrition and supplements may help to prevent attacks. It may be useful to take a small dose (0.5g) of the essential amino acid L-lysine, plus a vitamin B-complex.*

### Caution

*Shingles that affects the eye may cause serious complications and should be monitored carefully by your doctor.*

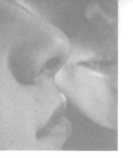

# Herpes simplex:
## cold sores

*An itchy or sore area, usually around the mouth or nose; a cluster of small blisters, which may ooze clear fluid before crusting over.*

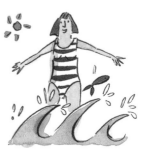

**T**hese unsightly, uncomfortable skin eruptions, which are caused by the *Herpes simplex* virus, may be the result of a cold, but are always triggered by stress – physical or emotional. Women often get cold sores during their periods; holiday-makers when exposed to too much sun.

### 🌐 Call the doctor

*If you suffer from recurrent herpes.*

**BELOW** Cold sores are not serious but can make you feel uncomfortable and miserable.

### ✚ CONVENTIONAL MEDICINE

Creams containing antiviral drugs may limit minor outbreaks, if used early. Antiviral tablets help prevent frequent recurrences and limit severe attacks.

**DOSAGE: ADULTS** Take antiviral tablets up to five times a day for 5 days; follow medical advice. Creams may need more frequent application.

**DOSAGE: CHILDREN** Follow medical advice given for tablets. Apply creams every few hours.

### 🌿 HERBAL REMEDIES

Tea-tree oil, oil of cade (a juniper extract), lavender oil, clove oil, *Aloe vera* sap, sliced garlic and house-leek juice can all help.

**USE AND DOSAGE** Capsules containing echinacea (up to 600mg daily) or golden seal (up to 100mg daily) help combat the infection.

Internally, lemon-balm tea can be effective.

### ✿ HOMEOPATHIC REMEDIES

**Natrum muriaticum 6c**

For pearly-white cold sores. May have mouth ulcers too. Swelling and burning of lower lip. Dry mouth and lips. Cracks in middle lower lip.

**DOSAGE** 1 tablet every 4 hours. Maximum 1 week.

# The Nervous System

The nervous system is an ultra-complex organization of nerves that carries impulses throughout the body, from organs such as the ears and eyes, skin and joints, to the brain. This delicate system is easily upset, leading to fatigue, stress, headaches and insomnia. However, many of these ailments may be greatly assisted by simple home remedies. Food, for example, has long been seen as nourishment not only for the body but also for the mind, while aromatherapy – smell being the most primitive of our senses – has a direct effect on the brain.

# Neuralgia

*Pain that is experienced like a knife or electric shock, often felt on one side of the face, where the trigeminal nerve is affected (trigeminal neuralgia); it may then settle down into a continual ache; other parts of the body are also vulnerable.*

**N**euralgia is pain in the nervous tissue, usually felt at the ends of the system – that is, near the surface of the skin. The most common forms are post-herpetic neuralgia (which often follows a bout of shingles; see *p.22*) and trigeminal neuralgia. These can both be so excruciating that washing, shaving and even the weight of bedclothes may be unbearable. In the treatment of neuralgia home remedies are not hugely successful, but neither are the very powerful drugs that are normally prescribed. The best chance of success comes from a combination of orthodox treatment, acupuncture and self-help.

**BELOW** Neuralgia can be stinging pain, soreness, tingling or numbness.

## ✚ CONVENTIONAL MEDICINE

Warmth or massage may help during an attack. Pain relievers may not be sufficient to control the pain, and your doctor may prescribe drugs used in other patients to treat depression or epilepsy. In intractable cases your doctor can refer you to a pain clinic, where a specialist may recommend a combination of different treatments, including behavioural therapy and acupuncture.

DOSAGE: ADULTS 1–2 tablets of pain relievers at onset of pain, repeated every 4 hours; consult pack.
DOSAGE: CHILDREN Give regular doses of liquid pain reliever; consult pack, or follow medical advice.

## ▱ HERBAL REMEDIES

One simple remedy is to smooth a little warmed lemon juice or diluted lemon oil on the painful area. Cayenne creams and infused oil are also useful externally, especially if the pain follows shingles; internally herbs to help repair nerves can be useful.
USE AND DOSAGE Drink a combination of St John's wort, vervain and camomile (equal amounts, 2tsp of the mix per cup), or try valerian, which is most easily used in tincture or tablets.

## NUTRITION

Eat plenty of potatoes, liver (but not if you are pregnant), nuts and seeds, brown rice, brazil nuts, milk, eggs, poultry, wholemeal bread, dried fruit, green and root vegetables, pulses and fish for their B vitamins, which are essential in the diet of neuralgia sufferers. If chewing is painful, make some soup from a wide variety of the foods containing the B vitamins, so that it can be drunk from a cup or, if this is easier, through a thick straw. Old-fashioned, home-made chicken soup that is enriched with Marmite, barley and brown rice offers a simple, nutritious and delicious way of providing them.

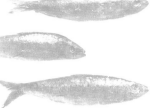

**ABOVE** All types of fish contain the essential B vitamins.

## HOMEOPATHIC REMEDIES

Spigelia 6c
For left-sided pain, like hot needles, sharp. Pain above left eye – person can point to the spot. Pain worse for stooping or opening mouth

Causticum 6c
For right-sided facial neuralgia. Worse for wind and for change of weather. Pain in jaws, worse for opening mouth.

Aconite 6c
For use in first stages. Intense pain after going out in cold, dry wind. Often left sided. May have tingling and numbness.

DOSAGE 1 tablet hourly for six doses, then every 4–6 hours. Maximum 3 days.

**Caution**

*Do not use rosemary oil if you have high blood pressure.*

## AROMATHERAPY

Lavender *(Lavandula angustifolia)*
Roman camomile *(Chamaemelum nobile)*
Marjoram *(Origanum majorana)*
Rosemary *(Rosmarinus officinalis)*
These oils are calming and soothing and help to ease the pain and tension of neuralgia.

APPLICATION They are best used in a cold compress held over the affected area. Do be aware that neuralgia is aggravated by stress *(see p.36)*, so find an anti-stress oil that you can use in the bath, as well as using the above oils on the specific area.

ROSEMARY

# Headaches

*Headache all over the scalp, with pain in the neck and shoulder muscles – likely causes: stress, tension, poor posture; frontal headache – likely causes: eyestrain, sinusitis; throbbing one-sided headache with nausea – likely cause: migraine.*

**H**eadaches are one of the most common reasons for consulting a doctor, yet they are rarely a symptom of any underlying disease. Though they frequently accompany acute infections, many routine headaches are mechanical in origin. Stress, anxiety, poor posture, badly designed work stations and the ever-growing use of computers can all result in tension developing in the neck and shoulders: by far the most common cause of everyday headaches.

## Caution

*Always read pain-reliever packages carefully, and do not exceed the stated dose.*

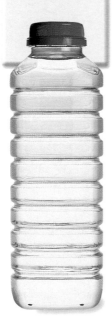

**LEFT** Boost your intake of fluids if you are prone to headaches.

### ➕ CONVENTIONAL MEDICINE

Drink plenty of water. Have a warm bath to relieve the tension. Rest in a quiet, darkened room and take a pain reliever.

**DOSAGE: ADULTS** 1–2 tablets of pain reliever at onset of pain, then every 4 hours; consult pack for details.

**DOSAGE: CHILDREN** Give regular doses of liquid pain reliever; consult pack, or follow medical advice.

### NUTRITION

Headaches can be triggered by low blood sugar levels. Eat at least some wholemeal toast and a banana for breakfast. Always have a banana and a bag of nuts and dried fruit to nibble on throughout the day. Beware of sudden drastic changes in your eating patterns; very low-calorie diets will also cause headaches, as will excessive alcohol and caffeine. A low fluid intake is one of the most common causes of headaches. Drink at least 1l/1¾pt of water every day, as well as other drinks. And it is important to differentiate between ordinary headaches and migraine (see p.30).

### HERBAL REMEDIES

There are various relaxing herbs for headaches.
USE AND DOSAGE Tension headaches often respond to betony and skullcap tea (1tsp of each per cup).

Use rosemary or a low dose of Korean ginseng (200mg daily) for headaches associated with overexertion and tiredness.

For headaches with depression use a combination of oats and vervain (1tsp of each per cup).

Lavender is good for burning headaches – use a few drops of tincture neat on the tongue or drink an infusion.

### AROMATHERAPY

- Lavender *(Lavandula angustifolia)*
- Peppermint *(Mentha x piperita)*
- Eucalyptus *(Eucalyptus radiata)*
- Basil *(Ocimum basilicum)*

Lavender is calming, soothing and a natural painkiller. Peppermint and basil clear the head. Eucalyptus clears the sinuses.
APPLICATION Put onto a facecloth with some cool water and use as a compress. For headaches due to a cold, put one drop of neat lavender on the tips of your fingers and massage into the temples, or a steam inhalation with eucalyptus will help. A couple of drops of basil on a handkerchief or on the pillow at night calms an overactive brain.

### HOMEOPATHIC REMEDIES

- Bryonia 30c

For pressing, bursting or splitting headache over left eye. Pain worse for least movement (even of the eye), for light, cough or stooping. Better for pressure.

- Nux vomica 30c

For splitting headache, sore scalp, dizziness, 'hangover' headache. Better for warmth, lying down. Worse for movement, draughts. Person is irritable and oversensitive.

DOSAGE 1 tablet every 4 hours, as needed. Maximum six doses.

### Call the doctor

*If the headache is the result of a blow to the head; if there is numbness, confusion or sudden drowsiness; if you have a headache and fever together with pain on bending forward, stiff neck or nausea, or a dislike of bright light; if a very severe headache starts suddenly; if your balance, speech, memory or vision is affected; if you wake up with headaches that are worse when you cough or sneeze.*

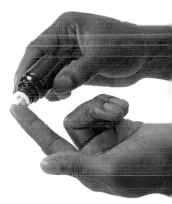

**ABOVE** A dab of lavender oil on the fingertips can be massaged into the temples for relief from many types of headache.

# Migraine

*Severe headache, which often starts with distorted vision; pain is frequently throbbing, on one side of the head, near an eye, and associated with nausea or vomiting; there may be pins and needles or weakness during an attack.*

**t is common for people who suffer from regular headaches to describe them as migraines. Sadly, there is no mistaking a real migraine, with its visual disturbances, nausea, violent vomiting and blinding pain. There is now a wide variety of drug treatments, but self-help may be the best long-term key to success. The saddest thing about migraine is that it becomes as much a social as a medical problem. Migraines are far more common in women than in men, especially around their periods: they tend to start after puberty and may improve after the menopause. It is common for migraine to run in families.**

**ABOVE AND BELOW** Watch your diet to spot any foods or drinks that trigger your migraine.

## CONVENTIONAL MEDICINE

Take soluble pain relief combined with an anti-emetic from your doctor. Modern prescription medicines may be able to avert an attack. Lie down in a darkened room, if possible, and drink plenty of water.

DOSAGE: ADULTS 1–2 tablets of pain reliever at onset of pain, repeated every 4 hours; consult pack.

DOSAGE: CHILDREN Give regular doses of liquid pain reliever; consult pack, or follow medical advice.

## NUTRITION

Naturopaths have known for decades that there is a link between migraine and food. The most common triggers are chocolate, citrus fruit, cheese and caffeine, though red and fortified wine, yeast extracts, pickled herrings, sauerkraut and other fermented foods are also thought to be causes. Many of these contain the chemical tyramine, which irritates blood vessels in the brain. Two or three glasses of cold water straight from the tap at the very earliest signs of a migraine may be enough to abort an attack, while ginger tea (see *Motion Sickness* on p.184) can help prevent vomiting, but it must be taken at the first sign of an attack.

### HERBAL REMEDIES

Lavender and betony are useful migraine herbs.
USE AND DOSAGE Combine equal amounts of both herbs in an infusion and then sip while the pain of a migraine continues.

Add 10 drops of feverfew tincture to a little water and take at 15-minute intervals during a migraine attack.

An equal amount of valerian tincture (a strong sedative) can also help.

### AROMATHERAPY

- Lavender *(Lavandula angustifolia)*
- Melissa *(Melissa officinalis)*
- Peppermint *(Mentha x piperita)* [if the migraine is accompanied by nausea and sickness]

Lavender is calming, soothing and a natural painkiller. Peppermint clears the head and stimulates the brain. Melissa is antidepressive and gently sedative.

APPLICATION Put the oil onto a facecloth with some cool water and use as a compress on the forehead or at the back of the neck. You can either add peppermint or melissa to the lavender or use them separately. Alternatively, put a drop of neat lavender on the tips of your fingers and massage well into the temples.

### HOMEOPATHIC REMEDIES

It is often best to consult a qualified homeopath for the treatment of migraine.

- Iris 30c

For blurred vision, then right-sided headache with nausea. Better for gentle motion. Often occurs at weekends.

- Sanguinaria 30c

For pulsating headache, beginning at back of head and extending to right eye. Better for vomiting, being asleep. Worse for light, noise, fasting. Starts in morning, improving during the day.

DOSAGE 1 tablet every 30 minutes until improved. Maximum six doses.

PEPPERMINT

**Caution**

*Avoid feverfew if taking prescribed blood-thinning drugs such as warfarin or heparin, as it can reduce the blood's clotting ability still further.*

**Prevention**

*Keep a detailed food and drink diary for at least 3 weeks. Then go back and identify foods eaten up to 3 hours before an attack. This will guide you towards foods that you should eliminate from your diet.*

# Fatigue

*Characterized by either mental or physical exhaustion; sleeping for longer than usual and waking feeling tired; an inability to concentrate and difficulty in summoning up the effort to rectify the problem.*

Extreme fatigue, or **TAT (Tired All the Time syndrome)**, has become a problem of almost epidemic proportions in Britain and the **US**, but it should not be confused with chronic fatigue syndrome or **ME** *(Myalgic encephalomyelitis, see p.34)*, in which fatigue is just one symptom of a complex illness. It is important to rule out the presence of any underlying illness, such as anaemia, thyroid problems, diabetes or glandular fever. In the absence of a more specific diagnosis, extreme fatigue is most likely to be caused by poor nutrition, insomnia *(see p.38)*, snoring, sleep apnoea, anxiety or depression.

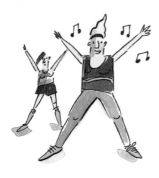

## ✚ CONVENTIONAL MEDICINE

Try to sleep regularly for 8–9 hours a night. Take regular exercise and eat a balanced diet, avoiding excessive alcohol. Consider taking some time out from domestic or paid employment. If symptoms persist for more than 2 weeks, see your doctor, who may arrange for some blood tests to rule out a physical cause for your symptoms.

## NUTRITION

A full complement of the many essential nutrients is the first requirement and this can only be achieved by a well-balanced diet. Rich sources of iron, like liver (but not if you are pregnant), other offal, dates, raisins, watercress, eggs, dark green leafy vegetables and sardines, must be top of your shopping list. Eat plenty of foods rich in vitamin C alongside the iron-rich foods to improve absorption – tomatoes with the sardines, orange juice with your boiled eggs.

Avoid all the commercial energy drinks, and do not go overboard on protein. What you need are starchy foods – but not biscuits, cakes and confectionery. Go for a small steak, plenty of potatoes (not always chips) and lots of vegetables or salad; a

### 🌑 Call the doctor
*If your symptoms have been present for more than 2 weeks.*

large portion of pasta with a little Bolognese sauce; or a selection of vegetables and a little chicken. It is important to keep blood sugar levels on a constantly even keel, and this can be best achieved by eating little and often: good-quality starchy food at least every 3 hours. Nuts, seeds, cereals and dried fruits are excellent sources of energy.

### HERBAL REMEDIES

Herbal tonics can be extremely effective in boosting energy levels to combat fatigue.

USE AND DOSAGE Korean ginseng (600mg daily) is extremely popular but can prove too stimulating for many – traditionally it should be used only by older age groups (40-plus), American ginseng or codonopsis is gentle; women may prefer Dang Gui.

Take Siberian ginseng (600mg daily) during busy times to help cope with additional stresses.

ABOVE Boost your starch intake, but ensure that you make healthy choices.

### AROMATHERAPY

- Rosemary (Rosmarinus officinalis)
- Lemon grass (Cymbopogon citratus)
- Basil (Ocimum basilicum)
- Peppermint (Mentha x piperita)

For mental fatigue, rosemary, basil and peppermint stimulate the brain. Lemon grass builds up the body's resistance to fatigue, and gives an energy boost.

APPLICATION Use these oils in the bath, in massage oils or lotions, in vaporizers or on a handkerchief.

### HOMEOPATHIC REMEDIES

A consultation with a qualified homeopath is recommended for fatigue.

- Nux vomica 30c

For competitive, ambitious workaholic, who becomes exhausted from overwork or overindulgence.

- Sepia 30c

Often used for the worn-out, weepy woman. Feels distant from family. Depressed and dislikes company. Feels the cold easily. May be better for exercise.

DOSAGE 1 tablet twice daily. Maximum 5 days.

**Prevention**

*Regular supplementation with zinc and a daily iron supplement should be routine for anyone on antidepressants or tranquillizers. Co-enzyme Q10 is another link in the conversion of food-to-energy chain and should also be taken every day.*

LEFT Basil oil is a good mental stimulant.

# Chronic fatigue syndrome: ME

*Fatigue from a particular date onwards; unexplained muscle weakness, often with painful joints or muscles, forgetfulness and difficulty in concentrating, mood swings and depression.*

Whole volumes have been written about **ME (myalgic encephalo-myelitis)** and some medical experts still believe that it is wholly a psychological illness. Typified by grinding fatigue and exhaustion, an inability to stay awake, muscle pains, mood swings and loss of concentration, enthusiasm and appetite – all of which can lead to severe depression – it is generally a poorly treated illness. The only route to long-term success is to combine treatment with self-help and the support of family and friends. Healthy eating is the foundation of recovery, and extreme dietary regimes of any sort should be avoided at all costs.

## 🌐 Call the doctor

*If symptoms of chronic fatigue syndrome persist.*

## ✚ CONVENTIONAL MEDICINE

Because the cause of ME is not known, there is no specific conventional remedy that has been shown to be more effective than any other. Most doctors recommend taking gentle, graded exercise, with rest periods when the symptoms are particularly severe. Eat a healthy diet. Take measures to limit stress, and consider undergoing counselling.

## ▢ HERBAL REMEDIES

Herbal immune stimulants, such as echinacea and astragalus, can help in the long term, while tonic herbs (such as ginseng, damiana or gotu kola) will provide an energy boost in the recovery stage, but taking them too soon can exhaust the system further.
USE AND DOSAGE Use drop doses of bitters, like wormwood or gentian tinctures, before meals to improve the digestion.

An infusion using equal amounts of vervain, betony and oatstraw can help with depression.

A daily bowl of shiitake mushroom soup acts as an immune tonic and restorative.

Take 1g of evening primrose oil daily as a nutritional supplement.

## NUTRITION

Do not leave more than 3 hours between eating, and eat natural-sugar foods like dried fruits when you need a boost. Take a daily high-dose multivitamin and mineral supplement.

Eat plenty of brown rice, wholemeal bread and pasta, and potatoes for their energy; liver, all the pulses and dark green vegetables for their B vitamins; citrus fruit, salads and vegetables for their vitamin C. Avoid alcohol, all caffeine, sugar, confectionery and any foods that have a poor nutritional value.

**ABOVE** Spinach is full of iron and chlorophyll, as well as B vitamins.

## AROMATHERAPY

The oils you choose depend on your symptoms:
FOR MUSCULAR FATIGUE:

- Thyme *(Thymus vulgaris)*
- Lemon grass *(Cymbopogon citratus)*
- Marjoram *(Origanum majorana)*

FOR INSOMNIA *(SEE ALSO P.38)*:

- Valerian *(Valeriana fuurlei)*
- Roman camomile *(Chamaemelum nobile)*

FOR DEPRESSION:

- Neroli *(Citrus aurantium)*
- Rose *(Rosa centifolia/Rosa damascena)*

The oils for muscular fatigue and insomnia are soothing and warming; those for depression are both warming to the mind and uplifting.

APPLICATION Use in baths, foot spas, for massage and in inhalations. Professional help from an aromatherapist can see you through this problem.

### Prevention

The general consensus is that ME is caused by a viral infection, so the only preventative measure may be maintenance of an adequate and efficient immune system.

## HOMEOPATHIC REMEDIES

- Carbolic acid 6c

For mental and physical fatigue. Very sensitive sense of smell. Band-like headaches. Belching and nausea. Craves stimulants.

- Calcarea carbonica 6c

For chilly, sweaty head, especially at night. Hard-working, conscientious, takes on too much, practical. Lots of sore throats.

DOSAGE 1 tablet daily. Maximum 2 weeks.

**ABOVE** Valerian makes a soothing oil for those suffering from ME.

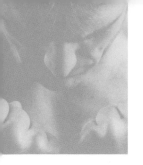

# Stress

*Typified by lots of minor medical ailments, often all at the same time, and possibly including a fast heartbeat; diarrhoea; an edgy or depressed feeling; difficulty sleeping; poor or increased appetite; irritability or tetchiness.*

I t is most important to realize that some stress is an essential ingredient of everyday life. What varies is the way in which people cope with different levels of stress. Once you have learned the levels you can comfortably withstand, it is not difficult to learn the skills needed to cope with higher stress levels. Whatever causes your stress, your body's response is the same. Large amounts of adrenalin are poured into your system, preparing you for 'flight or fight'. Difficulties arise when you cannot do either. In most cases counselling, psychotherapy and relaxation techniques can help, but home remedies play a major part, too.

## 🌑 Call the doctor

*If you have been feeling consistently stressed for more than 2 weeks.*

## ✚ CONVENTIONAL MEDICINE

Following a stressful episode, try to reorganize events to avoid further upset. Eat regular meals and take regular exercise – consider yoga or meditation relaxation therapy. Try to avoid resorting to alcohol or cigarettes. If the symptoms become unmanageable, your doctor may be able to make a referral to a counsellor. Drugs to control the symptoms or lift your mood are not a panacea, but may improve the symptoms to a point at which you are more able to help yourself.

## HERBAL REMEDIES

Relaxing herbs like betony, lemon balm, lavender, camomile, vervain or skullcap make ideal teas to soothe tensions and nervous stress. Valerian is sometimes referred to as 'nature's tranquillizer', so it is ideal for easing tensions: the taste is distinctive, so tablets may be preferable.

USE AND DOSAGE Use 1–2tsp of the relaxing herbs per cup of tea.

Siberian ginseng will help the body cope with stress: take 600mg daily in the week before expected stresses occur.

## ❋ HOMEOPATHIC REMEDIES

A consultation with a qualified homeopath is recommended for cases of stress.

🐚 **Nux vomica 30c**

For a competitive, impatient, ambitious go-getter. Symptoms of abdominal pain, which is cramping. Likes coffee, spices, alcohol and fats. Stress from overwork at the office.

**DOSAGE** I tablet twice daily. Maximum 5 days.

## 🍎 NUTRITION

It is hard to over-emphasize the role of nutrition in helping to calm a stressful life. Serotonin and tryptophan both have a calming effect on mind and body. For serotonin, eat plenty of nuts (especially walnuts), dates, figs, pineapples, pawpaws, passion fruit, tomatoes, avocados and aubergines. For tryptophan, eat plenty of potatoes, beans, pasta, rice and wholemeal bread. Porridge and muesli make a good start to the day. Get your protein from modest amounts of fish, poultry and low fat dairy products, as well as beans and cereals. The B vitamins and iron are also key requirements in a stressful life. Use herbs like rosemary, thyme, lemon balm, basil, lemon verbena, marjoram and nutmeg lavishly for their calming effects. Avoid excessive consumption of mental irritants, like alcohol and the caffeine in cola drinks, coffee, tea and chocolate.

## 💧 AROMATHERAPY

The range of potential oils is vast, so pick ones whose aroma you like: perhaps lavender, geranium, patchouli, clary sage or petitgrain; any of the citrus oils; the floral oils – niaouli, rose, jasmine, ylang ylang; woody oils such as sandalwood or cedarwood; vetivert. If your stress is a digestive, muscular or menstrual problem, look under those ailments.

**APPLICATION** Try not to make a regime for yourself that creates even more stress. Put the oil in the bath, in a burner, into a massage oil or body lotion, and just enjoy the pleasure of it.

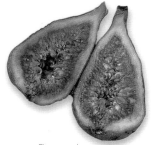
**ABOVE** Figs contain serotonin, which can calm the mind and body.

### Prevention

Planning your life to minimize over commitment and learning to say 'no' are the first steps in prevention. Yoga, meditation, relaxation exercises, massage and calming baths may all help.

COFFEE BEANS

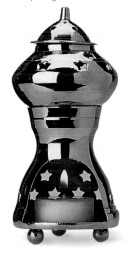
**BELOW** An aromatherapy burner is simple to use but reaps huge benefits.

# Insomnia

*Difficulty getting to sleep, which may occur at any time during normal sleeping hours.*

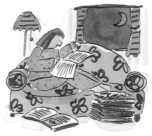

**N**one of us can escape the occasional bad night's sleep. Real insomnia, however, is a state of habitual sleeplessness, repeated night after night, often for months or even years on end. Worrying about insomnia, to the point of obsession, does more damage than the lack of sleep itself. But in most instances better sleep hygiene and a wealth of home remedies can help you get the sleep of the just.

**BELOW** Taking exercise during the day will help you sleep at night.

### CONVENTIONAL MEDICINE

Stop working at least an hour before bedtime. Have a hot milky drink and a bath (but not too hot). Avoid alcohol. Go to bed, but if you are awake after 30 minutes, get up and settle into a relaxing activity, such as reading a newspaper or magazine. After 30 minutes go back to bed. Repeat as many times as necessary. During the day (never just before bedtime), take regular aerobic exercise, at least three times a week. Seek medical advice if the symptoms of insomnia persist.

### HERBAL REMEDIES

A simple remedy suitable for all ages is Californian poppy, which can be grown in the garden as an annual and is an effective sleep-inducing remedy, with no potent side-effects.

USE AND DOSAGE Use Californian poppy fresh or dried in an infusion.

Also worth trying are passion flower, lavender and betony – use in equal amounts in an infusion as a night-time drink.

Cowslip flowers are a traditional and effective remedy for insomnia associated with overexcitement. Use a tincture and take 20–40 drops in hot milk before bed.

## NUTRITION

Going to bed too full or too hungry interferes with your normal sleep habits and thus leads to insomnia. Eating too late – especially a meal based on animal protein – is a great mistake, as such foods trigger greater production of the activity hormones. Evening meals should be based on starchy foods such as rice, pasta, potatoes, root vegetables and beans, saving meat meals for the middle of the day.

Eat plenty of offal (but not liver if you are pregnant), fish, poultry, eggs, potatoes, brown rice, wholegrain cereals, wholemeal bread and soya products, which are the best sources of vitamin $B_6$, lack of which can be a factor in insomnia. Culinary herbs can also be a tremendous help, especially sage, fennel, rosemary and basil.

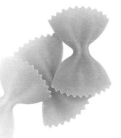

**ABOVE** An evening meal centred on pasta will satisfy your hunger.

## AROMATHERAPY

- Lavender (*Lavandula angustifolia*)
- Clary sage (*Salvia sclarea*)
- Orange (*Citrus aurantium/Citrus sinensis*)
- Marjoram (*Origanum majorana*)
- Basil (*Ocimum basilicum*)

These oils are calming and soothing. Basil helps to clear the mind; marjoram is a warming muscle-relaxant.

**APPLICATION** Use in a warm bath, or put a couple of drops on the pillow, in a burner or a light ring in the bedroom. Use the oils in combinations and find the aromas you like best.

## HOMEOPATHIC REMEDIES

- **Passiflora 30c**
For restless, wakeful sleep. Try this remedy first.
- **Nux vomica 30c**
For overworked person, who wakes in early hours thinking of work. Falls asleep just before time to wake up. Wakes with hungover feeling.
- **Coffea 30c**
For waking in early hours, mind full of ideas, dozing afterwards. Wakes suddenly, dreams disturb sleep.
**DOSAGE** 1 tablet taken before bed for 10 days or until improved.

### Caution

*Avoid sleeping tablets, which are addictive. They may be suitable for short-term treatment under medical supervision. Never drink alcohol or drive if you are using clary sage oil. It is very sedative and combines badly with alcohol.*

### Prevention

*A regular sleep routine is vital and depends on going to bed and getting up at roughly the same time every day – insomnia is quite rare in those who have to be up at 6am. Do not allow yourself to sleep during the day, as this will make getting back to normal even more difficult.*

# Seasonal affective disorder: SAD

*BASIL*

*Characterized by mood changes related to the seasons; it is often associated with a craving for carbohydrates, lethargy and insomnia.*

When the retina at the back of the eye is stimulated by light, the pineal gland is affected and the amount of the hormone melatonin circulating in the body is reduced. During the winter months there is not much sunlight, so more melatonin is released. Some people are much more severely affected by this lack of daylight than others and become extremely depressed.

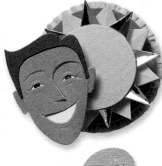

## CONVENTIONAL MEDICINE

Exposure to a bright light source for several hours a day can help in some cases.

## HERBAL REMEDIES

St John's wort and lemon balm are effective antidepressants. Basil is also very uplifting.

USE AND DOSAGE Eat plenty of fresh basil, and inhale the scent of the crushed leaves or put a few drops of the oil on a handkerchief.

Try taking 600mg of Siberian ginseng daily for 4–6 weeks in early winter.

## HOMEOPATHIC REMEDIES

This problem is complex to treat, so consult a qualified homeopath. The following remedies offer only a brief guide.

Sepia 30c

For person who cannot be bothered, even with family. Feels separated from them and depressed. Guilty feelings and tearful. Slow mentally and sharp-tongued. Better after exercise.

Aurum 30c

For depressed, sulky, weepy person. All emotions felt in the extreme. Critical of both self and others.

DOSAGE I tablet daily. Maximum 5 days.

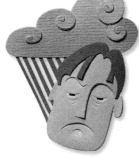

**ABOVE** Dramatic mood swings can make your life unbearable, but small lifestyle changes can make a big difference.

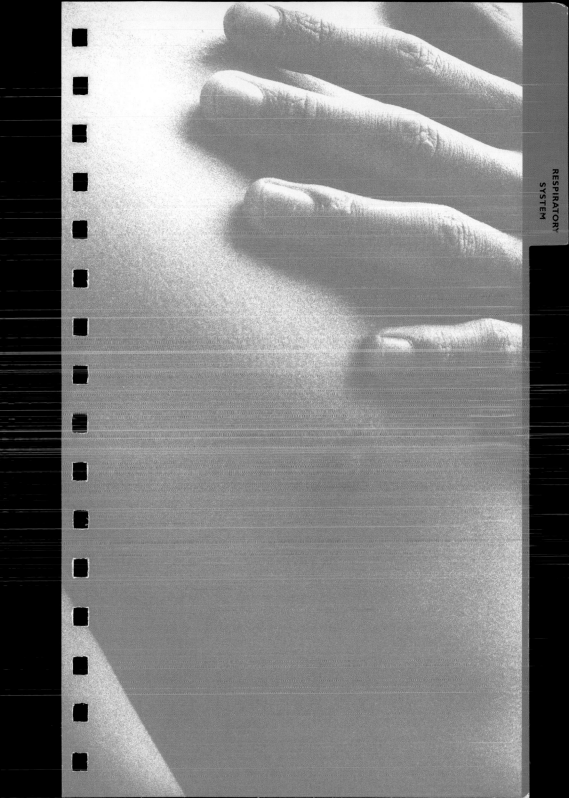

# The Respiratory System

Every minute we take approximately 12 breaths, drawing oxygen into our lungs and expelling carbon dioxide, but since this generally happens automatically we often ignore the respiratory system until something goes wrong with it. Viruses, irritation of the mucous membranes and inhaled pollutants can all threaten the respiratory tract, leading to coughs and colds, asthma and hay fever. This section suggests easy remedies to make these common ailments more bearable.

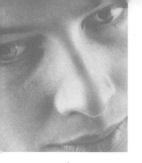

# Catarrh

*Typified by excessive amounts of thick mucus in the nose, throat and chest, which is caused by infection, allergy or irritation of the mucous membranes; plus a blocked or runny nose.*

rritation of the mucous membranes in the nose and throat, or allergic reactions, can cause an increase in the amount of mucus produced by these tissues. Viral or bacterial infections can also produce the same reaction and, if the sinuses become congested and infected, this can lead to sinusitis *(see p.50)*.

## Prevention

*Stop smoking and avoid exhaust fumes, chemical smells and other irritant pollutants. Avoid allergens* (see Allergies on p.14). *Blow your nose often to reduce the risk of infection.*

### CONVENTIONAL MEDICINE

Catarrh will improve without any treatment, usually within a week or two. However, steam inhalations *(see p.196)* make the mucus thinner and breathing more comfortable, and help to reduce the swelling; they can be used as often as necessary. Decongestants can help too, particularly ones that are sprayed up the nose. Beware: if continued for more than a week, a nasal decongestant will actually make the nose more stuffy than it was before.

DOSAGE: ADULTS AND CHILDREN  Most nasal decongestants should be sprayed into the nose at least twice a day.

### HERBAL REMEDIES

A combination of astringent and soothing herbs will help clear catarrh and ease inflamed membranes.

USE AND DOSAGE  Try mixing equal amounts of dried elderflower, eyebright, marsh-mallow leaves and ribwort plantain, then use in infusions (2tsp to a cup of boiling water, four times a day).

Steam inhalants can also help. Mix 5 drops each of sandalwood and eucalyptus oils with 5ml/1tsp of friar's balsam (compound tincture of benzoin) in a basin of boiling water and then inhale for 10 minutes. If you have a eucalyptus tree in your garden, use a handful of fresh leaves steeped in boiling water instead.

### AROMATHERAPY

- Eucalyptus *(Eucalyptus radiata)*
- Benzoin *(Styrax benzoin)*
- Basil *(Ocimum basilicum)*
- Thyme *(Thymus vulgaris)*

These oils relieve congestion and help to fight infection. But if catarrh is due to an allergy *(see p.14)*, then lavender or camomile may be more beneficial.

APPLICATION Steam inhalation and/or facial massage from a therapist for specific pressure points are generally beneficial.

### HOMEOPATHIC REMEDIES

There are many catarrh remedies *(see also Sinusitis on p.50)*. If the following do not help, then consult a homeopath.

- Kali bichromicum 6c

For thick, ropy, gluey, green or yellow catarrh. Pressing pain in root of nose. Dry crusts in nose. Worse for hot weather.

- Pulsatilla 6c

For stuffed-up nose, white/yellow-green discharge. Better in open air. Loss of smell or foul smell in nose from catarrh. Ears may discharge.

- Sambucus nigra 6c

For snuffles in babies, with difficulty suckling.

DOSAGE 1 tablet every 4 hours until condition improves. Maximum 12 doses.

### NUTRITION

Naturopaths believe that a high consumption of dairy products can increase the production of mucus. So cut down on all milk-based foods for a couple of weeks. If you do this for any longer, get professional guidance about your diet and about supplements, to prevent calcium and other deficiencies.

Eat plenty of onions, chives, spring onions, leeks and garlic, all traditional foods for the relief of catarrh; sweet potatoes, carrots, broccoli and red or dark green cabbage for their beta-carotene. Be sure to add thyme, rosemary, ginger, chillis and horse-radish to recipes, as these are decongestants.

**Caution**

These oils (excluding the lavender and camomile) are all very strong and should probably not be used for small children.

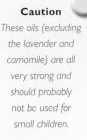

**BELOW** Leeks, chillis and ginger can all bring relief from catarrh.

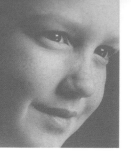

# Common cold

*Characterized by a fever; streaming nose; sneezing; tickly cough; and a sore throat; often accompanied by generalized muscular aches and pains, together with a lack of energy.*

There are hundreds of different viruses that are responsible for the symptoms of a cold, and coughing or sneezing in confined spaces may transmit the virus via infected mucus. The common cold has defied the combined efforts of all the world's doctors, virologists and other medical experts, and this is one condition for which the old wives' tales often produce the best results. So encourage your body's natural defences by taking plenty of rest, eating nutritiously and enjoying the benefits of steam treatment and other simple home remedies.

## Caution

*Always read pain-reliever packages carefully, and make sure that you do not exceed the stated dose.*

**BELOW** A cold may affect your sense of taste, but try to eat a balanced diet.

### ✚ CONVENTIONAL MEDICINE

Fever and malaise can be treated with pain relievers, which often need to be continued for several days until the symptoms subside. Inhalations of steam *(see p.196)* as often as possible help to clear the nasal passages and make breathing easier. Babies may need nose drops to enable them to breathe more easily while feeding. Colds usually last between 3 and 10 days.

DOSAGE: ADULTS 1–2 tablets of pain relievers at onset of fever, then every 4 hours; consult pack for details.

DOSAGE: CHILDREN Give regular doses of liquid pain reliever; consult pack, or follow medical advice.

### ◊ AROMATHERAPY

- Eucalyptus *(Eucalyptus radiata)*
- Tea tree *(Melaleuca alternifolia)*
- Pine *(Pinus sylvestris)*

Tea tree will make you sweat, which helps to eliminate the virus (make sure that you drink extra fluid). Eucalyptus and pine help to ease stuffiness; add lavender at night, to help you sleep.

APPLICATION Use these oils in vaporizers or inhalations (on handkerchiefs and bedcovers) to ease congestion. In a burner they help to reduce the risk of secondary infections. Or put them in the bath, using tea-tree oil at the first onset of symptoms.

### ❋ HOMEOPATHIC REMEDIES

**✍ Aconite 30c**

For first signs of cold. Frequent sneezing, nose bunged up. Thirsty, worse for stuffy rooms.

**✍ Allium cepa 30c**

For profuse sneezing, streaming eyes and nose. Hot, thirsty, better in fresh air. Nose sore.

**✍ Natrum muriaticum 30c**

For cold that begins with sneezing. Discharge from nose, like the white of an egg. Nose may also be blocked. Cold sores, mouth ulcers and cracked lips.
DOSAGE 1 tablet up to every 4 hours, as needed. Maximum 3–4 days.

### NUTRITION

Eat plenty of fresh fruit, salads and raw vegetables; at least two cloves of raw garlic daily (onions and garlic have a very powerful antiseptic and decongestant effect); thick onion soup or oven-baked onions daily. Drink plenty of fluids to replace those lost through sweating and sneezing, but stick mainly to fruit juices, plain water, herbal teas and a hot water, lemon and honey mixture. Avoid dairy products and all sugary food for 2 or 3 days.

### HERBAL REMEDIES

Herbs can ease many symptoms of a cold, and some display antiviral activity to combat the cause.
USE AND DOSAGE A tea that is made from equal parts of elderflower, peppermint (use catmint instead for children), yarrow and hyssop (1tsp per cup, taken up to four times daily) will ease catarrh, chills and coughs.

Gargling with a standard infusion of sage will soothe sore throats; you can improve the flavour with fresh lemon juice.

Take up to 10 × 200mg echinacea capsules daily, for up to 4 days, to boost the immune system.

### Prevention

*Eat plenty of pumpkin seeds, oysters and other shellfish to keep your zinc uptake up to the mark. When there are lots of colds around, suck 3 or 4 zinc and vitamin C lozenges each day to boost your immunity.*

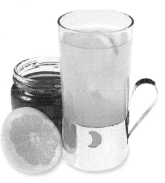

**ABOVE** A hot lemon and honey drink makes you feel better, as well as having nutritional benefits.

# Coughs and bronchitis

*The explosive release of air from the lungs, caused by inflammation of the bronchi, the larger air passages leading to the lungs; mucus that is clear or coloured, often yellow or brown; a dry, tickly throat.*

**A** cough may be due to nothing more than inhaled irritants like dust, exhaust fumes, smoke or a crumb of food. Of all symptoms in the respiratory tract, a cough is the commonest, but it may be a sign of underlying illness. Acute bronchitis, however, is caused by an infection, often following flu or a severe cold. Chronic bronchitis is known as the 'English disease', caused by repeated irritation from damp air and smoking, leading to an overproduction of mucus. This reduces the amount of oxygen available, making the heart work harder. A chest infection on top of chronic bronchitis causes severe breathing problems.

## 🌐 Call the doctor

*If you have a deep cough; if you are coughing up blood-stained mucus, which may be a sign of more serious illness.*

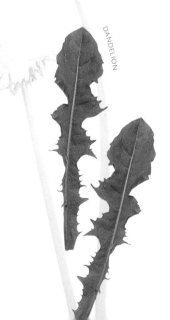

DANDELION

## ✚ CONVENTIONAL MEDICINE

A dry cough will often be relieved by a steam inhalation (see p.196), which you can have as often as necessary. If a cough does not clear up within 2–3 weeks, see your doctor. A deeper cough, such as the type that develops after a cold into bacterial lung infection (most common in children and the elderly) may require antibiotics. There is no evidence that cough medicines have any effect.

## ◻ NUTRITION

For all respiratory problems a daily bowl of garlic soup is invaluable, as it is both decongestant and antibacterial. Eat plenty of celery, parsley and fresh dandelion leaves (dandelion teabags are now available if you do not have a garden) to increase your urinary output and get rid of body fluids; onions and leeks (the same family as garlic); fish, pulses, brown rice and bananas for their B vitamins; liver, carrots, sweet potatoes and spinach for their vitamin A; oily fish for their anti-inflammatory properties. Cut out all salt in order to prevent fluid retention. Reduce your intake of all dairy products to help lessen mucus formation.

### HERBAL REMEDIES

Herbal cough remedies can ease bronchial spasms, expel phlegm, lubricate a dry cough or suppress an irritant one.

USE AND DOSAGE For chesty coughs or bronchitis, use thyme, elecampane, mullein, cowslip, white horehound or Iceland moss in teas (1tsp per cup) sweetened with honey.

A syrup can be made by layering slices of onion or turnip with sugar, leave overnight, then drink the liquid in 5ml/1tsp doses.

Cough suppressants like wild cherry can ease nervous, irritant coughs but should be avoided when trying to expel phlegm.

### HOMEOPATHIC REMEDIES

Rumex 6c

For throat tickling with cold air, spasmodic dry cough preventing sleep. Hoarseness. Phlegm tough, worse for talking and cold air. Better for covering the mouth.

Bryonia 6c

For dry, hacking, spasmodic cough. Must sit up. Worse for eating, drinking, at night. Cough on entering warm room. Holds chest on coughing.

DOSAGE 1 tablet three times daily until improved. Maximum 2 weeks.

### AROMATHERAPY

Sandalwood (Santalum album)

Benzoin (Styrax benzoin)

Eucalyptus (Eucalyptus radiata)

Frankincense (Boswellia sacra)

Tea tree (Melaleuca alternifolia)

Steam inhalations using these oils soothe the throat and airways, and assist in expelling excess mucus. Massage of the throat and chest eases the tension there, especially if you are coughing a lot. Gargling ensures that no infection sets in in the throat.

APPLICATION Use sandalwood, benzoin, eucalyptus or frankincense in steam inhalations. Massage the throat/chest with any of these; use tea tree for gargles.

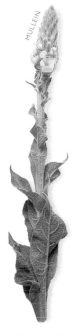

MULLEIN

**Prevention**

*Don't smoke; don't smoke; don't smoke. Avoid other smokers. Keep the lungs in good condition through regular exercise. Keep bedrooms cool and well aired and make sure that you wear a protective mask for all dusty DIY jobs and when air-pollution levels are high.*

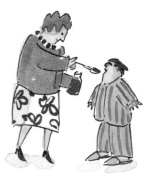

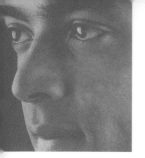

HONEY BE

# Hay fever

*Typified by repeated sneezing fits; either a
blocked or a constantly runny nose; sore, itchy
eyes, which may be inflamed; a tickle in the roof of
the mouth.*

**H**ay fever is an allergic reaction to the pollen produced by grasses
that mainly flower in the spring and summer. The sore, puffy eyes,
streaming nose and violent bouts of sneezing are instantly recogniz-
able. But it is not only grass pollens that cause hay fever – and today
the term is often used to describe allergic reactions to other airborne
irritants, like exhaust fumes, general atmospheric pollution and even
strong smells, like some perfumes. Some unfortunate people suffer
constantly from the symptoms – a condition known as perennial
rhinitis, most often caused by the droppings of the house dustmite.

## CONVENTIONAL MEDICINE

Drug treatments come as eyedrops, tablets and
nose sprays (do not use for more than 7 days).
**DOSAGE: ADULTS** Take most tablets once a day; eyedrops more often; consult pack, or follow medical
advice. Apply 2 puffs of spray per nostril twice a day.
**DOSAGE: CHILDREN** Doses of antihistamine syrup
depend on the age of the child; consult pack, or
follow medical advice. For children over 6 years,
apply 2 puffs of nose spray per nostril twice a day.

## HOMEOPATHIC REMEDIES

Hay fever can be treated by using mixed
pollens (30c taken once fortnightly
during the season). Homeo-
pathic tablets can be bought over the
counter; alternatively try one of the following:
**Allium cepa 6c**
For running, sore nose, watering but not sore eyes.
Worse for warm rooms. Better in the open air.
**Euphrasia 6c**
For watery and sore eyes, running but not sore
nose. Worse for light and warmth.
**DOSAGE** 1 tablet twice daily. Maximum 2 weeks.

### HERBAL REMEDIES

Herbalists often treat hay fever by using strengthening and cleansing herbs for the respiratory tract early on in the year, before the problem becomes too severe.

USE AND DOSAGE Make an infusion containing elderflower (3 parts), white horehound (2 parts), fumitory (1 part) and vervain (1 part), then drink 1–2 cups daily from late January until Easter.

To relieve symptoms that occur during the actual hay-fever season, take eyebright in capsules (up to 8 x 200mg daily) and bathe the eyes with either well-strained, sterilized marigold or eyebright infusions.

### AROMATHERAPY

᠊᠊ Roman camomile *(Chamaemelum nobile)*
᠊᠊ Basil *(Ocimum basilicum)*
᠊᠊ Melissa *(Melissa officinalis)*

Camomile and melissa are both anti-allergens; basil helps to clear the sinuses and the head of the nasty effects of hay fever.

APPLICATION Place 1 drop of each oil on a handkerchief, which you can then carry with you for instant relief. You can also use these oils for massaging the upper back and chest.

### NUTRITION

Reduce your intake of dairy produce – naturopaths believe this to be mucus-forming, which may exacerbate the problem. If this helps and you make permanent changes to your diet, make sure that you replace the missing nutrients (especially the calcium) from other sources. Vitamin C and its accompanying bioflavonoids are important protectors of the mucous membranes. All berries and fresh currants supply large quantities of both, and citrus fruit (including some of the pith and skin) should also be eaten in abundance.

If you have a pollen allergy, eating a couple of dessertspoons daily of honey made by bees feeding on flowers in your locality can provide great relief.

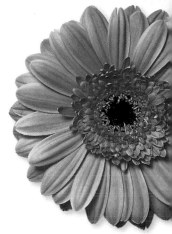

ABOVE Gently bathing the eyes in a flower infusion can bring relief from itchiness.

#### Prevention

*If you suffer from pollen allergy, stay indoors early in the morning and late in the evening, keep the windows closed and wear wrap around sunglasses.*

BELOW Strawberries contain a surprising amount of vitamin C.

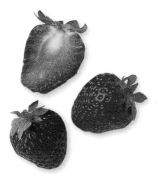

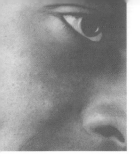

# Sinusitis

*Pain in the face or gums, a persistent headache, often over the eyes; pain worse on leaning forward; foul taste in the mouth; blood-stained discharge from the nose; completely or partially blocked nose.*

A heavy cold, allergies, irritant fumes, smoking, upper respiratory infections, nasal polyps or adverse reactions to some foods may all be the cause of sinusitis. This inflammation of the membranes lining the sinuses, and their consequent overproduction of mucus, is what produces the symptoms of headaches, facial pain, stuffiness, loss of smell, pain in the teeth, repeated episodes of chest and ear infections and thick, infected mucus. While antibiotics may be essential to treat severe infections, home remedies are best for milder conditions as well as for prevention.

**BELOW** Home remedies might need to be supplemented by antibiotic treatment for a severe or prolonged attack of sinusitis.

## CONVENTIONAL MEDICINE

Treatment depends on improving drainage from the sinus, together with treating the infection. Steam helps to make the mucus thinner and reduces nasal congestion. Nose sprays containing decongestants may help, but if used for too long can make the congestion worse. Antibiotics may be needed to clear the infection. Recurrent sinusitis may require surgical treatment.

## HERBAL REMEDIES

Anticatarrhal herbs, such as elderflower, camomile, ground ivy, coltsfoot, yarrow, eyebright or plantain can all help.

**USE AND DOSAGE** Make teas using 2tsp of herb per cup: add a pinch of golden seal or bayberry powder or 5 drops of tincture to the mix, if any of these are available.

Gently massaging the sinus areas with a cream or infused oil containing any of these herbs will also help alleviate sinusitis.

Add 10 drops each of eucalyptus, peppermint, pine and sandalwood oils to a basin of hot water and inhale for up to 10 minutes.

## ❋ HOMEOPATHIC REMEDIES

There are many remedies that help sinusitis. If these do not help, consult a qualified homeopath.

**Kali bichromicum 6c**

For thick, yellow, ropy catarrh. Pulsating pain at root of nose and frontal sinuses worse for stooping. Pressure in ear. Worse for cold, dry weather. Loss of smell.

**Hepar sulphuris calcareum 6c**

For thick, white or yellow, smelly mucus that makes nose sore. Person irritable. Facial bones sore. Right-sided shooting pains.

**Dosage** 1 tablet three times daily until improved. Maximum 10 days.

**ABOVE** Avoid dairy foods, but keep up your vitamin intake with plenty of fresh fruit and vegetables.

## ◖ NUTRITION

The food that most commonly increases the production of mucus, especially in children, is cow's milk, so try excluding cow's milk and milk products from your diet for a few weeks. If this does help and you are going to exclude them in the long term, make sure you get plenty of calcium and vitamin D from other sources (see Osteoporosis on p.70).

To maintain healthy sinuses, vitamins A, C and E and bioflavonoids are important, so eat plenty of carrots, apricots and dark green leafy vegetables; citrus fruit, with some of the pith and skin; dark cherries, tomatoes and mangoes; avocados, olive, sunflower and safflower oils. Garlic, horseradish, onions and leeks are all powerful weapons, while pineapple juice is healing: drink at least three glasses, diluted 50:50 with water, each day. Reduce your salt intake and go easy on the alcohol.

### Prevention

*For those who are susceptible to sinus problems, a monthly 2-day cleansing regime of nothing but raw fruit, vegetables and salads – as much as you like – with plenty of fruit and vegetable juices is a highly protective bonus.*

## ◖ AROMATHERAPY

**Basil** *(Ocimum basilicum)*
**Eucalyptus** *(Eucalyptus radiata)*
**Tea tree** *(Melaleuca alternifolia)*

These help to fight infection and clear the sinuses.

**Application** Put the oils on a handkerchief, in a burner, an electric vaporizer, a light ring or just a bowl of warm water. Steam inhalation is also effective.

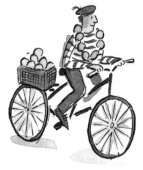

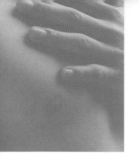

# Asthma

*Recurrent periods of difficulty in breathing; tightness in the chest, usually associated with a wheezing cough, particularly at night (this may be the only symptom to be apparent in children).*

A sthma is an extremely serious illness and can be life-threatening. The following home remedies must be taken in context with any advice given by your medical practitioner, but can greatly improve your quality of life and reduce the frequency and severity of asthma attacks. In recent years the incidence of asthma has dramatically increased – probably due to increasing amounts of atmospheric pollution, the growing addition of complex chemicals to food and drink, and the double glazing, insulation and draught-proofing of our homes. It most commonly affects children, but adults can suffer from late-onset asthma.

### 🌐 Call the doctor

*If you are already asthmatic but have noticed that you need more medication recently than usual; if there is a rapid deterioration in your condition.*

### CONVENTIONAL MEDICINE

Most asthmatics will already be taking prescribed medication, which will need to be increased when an attack starts. If you are experiencing your first asthma attack, seek urgent medical attention.

### HERBAL REMEDIES

Herbal antispasmodics and broncho-dilators are very effective in treating asthma – although the most potent herbs, such as ephedra and lobelia, are confined to professional use.

USE AND DOSAGE  For mild cases, a steam inhalant of camomile flowers (1tbsp to a basin of boiling water) can often avert an attack.

Macerate 2tsp of elecampane root overnight in a cup of cold water, then heat to boiling point; strain and sweeten with 1tsp of honey, then sip the liquid as required.

### HOMEOPATHIC REMEDIES

Asthma is a serious condition and may require medical attention. Do not stop medication from your doctor. It helps to consult a qualified homeo-path for this ailment.

### Caution

*Avoid non-steroidal anti-inflammatory drugs, such as ibuprofen or aspirin, which may make your asthma worse.*

### Arsenicum album 6c

For wheezing, anxiety, restlessness, fear of suffocation. Worse 1–3am, in cold air. Better for bending forward, warm drinks.

### Ipecacuanha 6c

For rattly chest, unable to cough up phlegm. Wheezy, chest feels tight. Cough with each breath. Nausea. Better for sitting up and in open air.

**DOSAGE** 1 tablet three times daily. Maximum period 1 week.

## NUTRITION

In children, asthma is usually an allergic response to inhaled allergens, but food and food additives can also be triggers. Keep a detailed food diary, noting when the attacks occur. This should give you some clues as to the foods that might be better avoided. Food additives like colourings, flavourings and preservatives can be severe triggers, while one of the most common food groups to cause problems is dairy foods, as milk and milk products tend to increase the body's production of mucus. You may need professional guidance to make sure that your child does not suffer nutritional deficiencies if you start excluding major foods.

A diet that is rich in all the protective antioxidants that are so important for the health of lung tissue is essential. Salads, grapes, melons, tomatoes, peppers, kiwis, wholegrain cereals and lots of all the green vegetables should be the basis of the asthmatic's diet.

**ABOVE** Eat plenty of salads for a diet rich in antioxidants.

### Caution

*Do not use frankincense in a steam inhalation, as the heat will increase the inflammation of the mucous membrane, making the congestion worse.*

## AROMATHERAPY

### Frankincense (Boswellia sacra)

Frankincense slows and deepens the breathing – it is used by monks when they are going into deep meditation. If asthma is an allergic reaction, try camomile instead (see also Stress on p.36).

**APPLICATION** Use in a vaporizer, compress or bath, or for localized massage around the chest/facial area. Frankincense can also be put on a tissue or pillow to help you breathe.

**BELOW** If you find dairy products make asthma attacks worse or more frequent, eliminate them from your diet.

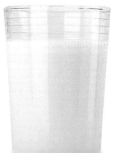

# Hiccups

*A sudden intake of breath, which is associated with a characteristic sound and sensation that are caused by a spasm of the diaphragm; often repeated several times before stopping.*

t is a sudden spasm of the diaphragm that causes a hiccup, triggered by irritation of the major nerve that supplies this muscle. Hiccups usually come in clusters and may last anything from a minute or so to hours, or even months. Attacks are nearly always the result of indigestion, overeating, rushing a meal or consuming lots of fizzy drinks, although occasionally they may be a sign of underlying and serious disease, such as liver abscess or kidney failure. Surprisingly, even medical textbooks suggest the traditional remedies of the cold key down the back or drinking from the wrong side of a glass.

**BELOW** Lie on your back with your knees bent.

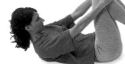

**BELOW** Bring up your knees and pull them towards your chest as hard as you can.

**BELOW** Hold for 3 seconds, then relax and repeat. This will stop the spasms that cause hiccups.

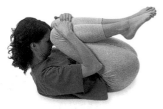

## ✚ CONVENTIONAL MEDICINE

If hiccups persist, consult your doctor, who may prescribe a drug to relax the diaphragm.

## ✿ HOMEOPATHIC REMEDIES

☙ **Cajup 6c**
For sudden attacks of hiccups at any provocation – talking, laughing, eating or motion.

☙ **Ignatia 6c**
For hiccups from emotional causes, when eating, drinking or smoking. Empty sensation in stomach.

☙ **Cyclamen 6c**
For hiccup-like burping. Worse for fatty food. Hiccups during pregnancy or while yawning.

☙ **Nux vomica 6c**
For hiccups from overeating or -drinking.
**DOSAGE** 1 tablet every 30 minutes until improved. Maximum 12 doses.

## ▭ HERBAL REMEDIES

See also flatulence and indigestion *(pp.86 and 80)*.
**USE AND DOSAGE** Sip peppermint or fennel infusion, or take 2–3 drops of cinnamon or clove oil on a lump of sugar. Eating pawpaw fruit or juice, or chewing crystallized ginger, can also help.

# The Circulatory System

**B**lood is pumped around the body by the heart at a rate of about 5l/10pt per minute, but if for any reason this blood flow is restricted, then circulatory problems – for instance, varicose veins, chilblains and restless legs – may result. If the blood has a reduced ability to absorb oxygen and convey it around the body, then anaemia may ensue. In both cases simple home remedies, combined with regular exercise to stimulate the entire cardiovascular system, can make a major difference. Circulatory problems are, however, easier to prevent than to cure.

# Anaemia

*Characterized by tiredness; pale skin; shortness of breath
on even mild exertion; rapid heart rate and palpitations;
swollen ankles; a feeling of faintness and generalized
symptoms of fatigue.*

**A**naemia is a condition in which the blood has a reduced ability to absorb oxygen and transport it around the body in the form of haemoglobin. Around 90 per cent of all cases are the result of iron deficiency, and heavy or prolonged periods, blood loss from ulcers, piles or gum disease are all likely causes. Many women of childbearing age are iron-deficient, but poor diet, deficiencies of folic acid and vitamin B$_{12}$, leukaemia, sickle cell anaemia and thalassaemia are comparatively rare causes. Vegetarians and pregnant women are vulnerable to anaemia. Dietary improvement is nearly always the answer.

### 🌐 Call the doctor

*If you think you are
suffering from anaemia.*

### ✚ CONVENTIONAL MEDICINE

Because there are several different types of anaemia, you should consult your doctor before taking any treatment. Often a course of iron tablets is all that is required, but some kinds of anaemia do not need any treatment, and iron may even make the condition worse. Your doctor may need to arrange for a blood test to be done before advising you. Pregnant women often need to take iron and folic acid supplements.

DOSAGE: ADULTS AND CHILDREN If you have iron deficiency, start with 1 iron tablet a day; see pack for details. Be aware that iron may causesconstipation.

### 🍎 NUTRITION

Always eat vitamin C-rich foods together with those containing iron, in order to improve absorption. Nettle soup and dandelion leaves added to salads are unusual but effective ways of getting lots of extra iron. You can also make both plants into tea, by adding 1tsp of chopped leaves to a cup of boiling water. Add parsley, chives, lovage, fennel, watercress and elderberries to salads and also to fruit dishes.

Eat plenty of offal for its vitamin $B_{12}$; meat, black pudding, green vegetables, watercress, pulses, wholegrain cereals, molasses, dried fruits, cashew nuts, wheatgerm, tomato purée, yeast extracts and brewer's yeast for their iron and folic acid. For vegetarians a traditional balti vegetable curry cooked in a cast-iron pot is an excellent source of iron that is well absorbed. In severe cases of anaemia, food sources are not sufficient and supplements will form an essential part of your recovery.

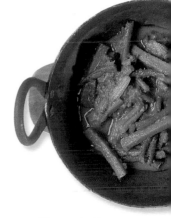

**ABOVE** Curry cooked in a cast-iron pot contains lots of easily absorbed iron.

## HERBAL REMEDIES

Those plants said to 'rob the soil' – such as stinging nettles and parsley – are especially rich in iron. Bitter herbs (like gentian) will improve the digestion and mineral absorption.

USE AND DOSAGE Make a tonic by steeping 100g/3½oz each of stinging nettle, Chinese angelica (Dang Gui) and dandelion root in 1l/1¾pt of red wine for 2 weeks; strain and drink one sherry glass per day.

Echinacea (2 × 200mg capsules daily) can help stimulate red blood-cell production.

## HOMEOPATHIC REMEDIES

The cause of anaemia should be established first. A consultation with a qualified homeopath, who may work in conjunction with your doctor, is suggested.

### Ferrum metallicum 6c

For person who appears strong, flushed, has cold hands and feet, but feels weak after any effort. Hammering headache. Flushes easily from pain or emotions. Ringing in the ears before periods. Anaemia due to heavy periods.

### Calcarea phosphorica 6c

For children who are growing rapidly. Anaemia after illness. Person dissatisfied with life and looking for something new. Tends to irritation.

### China 6c

For anaemia from blood loss. Feels weak, sensitive and nervous. Easily upset and feels chilly.

DOSAGE 1 tablet twice daily. Maximum 2 weeks.

### Prevention

*Eat well and regularly, including all the foods listed under Nutrition. Avoid restrictive weight-loss diets or any other nutritional regime that seems extreme.*

**BELOW** Parsley and wine both contain iron.

# Chilblains

*Painful, itchy, dark red swellings, which often affect the skin on the surface of the fingers and toes, but can also affect the ears, cheeks and nose; if serious, chilblains may begin to ulcerate.*

These sore, itching, inflamed and frequently swollen patches of skin occur most commonly on the backs of the fingers or tops of the toes. Sometimes they crop up on the ears, outer thighs and other parts of the body that are subject to cold and/or pressure. The cause is restriction of the circulating blood supply in the capillaries – the tiniest blood vessels at the very end of the system – leading to lack of oxygen and nutrients, and consequent cell damage. Prevention is the only cure.

### 🌐 Call the doctor

*If a chilblain begins to ulcerate.*

### ➕ CONVENTIONAL MEDICINE

Avoid chilblains by wrapping up warmly in cold weather. Several thinner layers can be more effective than one thick one. Once developed, a chilblain may take several weeks to recover. Take pain relievers if required.

DOSAGE: ADULTS 1–2 tablets of pain reliever at onset of pain, repeated every 4 hours; see pack for details.

DOSAGE: CHILDREN Give regular doses of liquid pain reliever; consult pack, or follow medical advice.

### 🔲 HERBAL REMEDIES

For habitual sufferers, circulation can be improved by teas containing prickly ash bark, ginger, cinnamon twigs or angelica root.

USE AND DOSAGE Simmer 1tsp of dried herb – either singly or in combination – with 2 cups of water for 10 minutes; add a pinch of cayenne powder before drinking.

Cayenne cream can help to ease discomfort, or try using compresses or foot baths containing oak-bark decoction.

Topical itching can be eased with arnica (do not use this, however, if the skin is broken), *Aloe vera* or marigold creams.

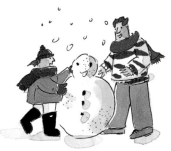

## NUTRITION

Increase your consumption of vitamin E by eating plenty of avocados, all nuts and seeds, and olive oil; buckwheat (added to bread, cake or biscuit recipes, or as pancakes) for its rutin content; citrus fruit, blackcurrants, cherries and blueberries for their vitamin C and bioflavonoids, which are essential nutrients for effective peripheral circulation. To prevent chilblains, take a daily dose of 400 IU of vitamin E and 1g of vitamin C with bioflavonoids. Also take a B complex that includes nicotinic acid.

One unit of alcohol per day for women (two for men) will help open up the tiniest blood vessels. But larger amounts have the opposite effect, making chilblains worse. Caffeine in any form is a vasoconstrictor and reduces blood supply, as does nicotine.

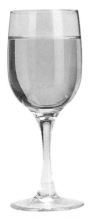

**ABOVE** A glass of white wine a day might open up tiny blood vessels and ease chilblains.

## AROMATHERAPY

- Geranium *(Pelargonium graveolens)*
- Black pepper *(Piper nigrum)*
- Lavender *(Lavandula angustifolia)*

These oils are warming, soothing, increase the circulation and have a slight painkilling effect.

**APPLICATION** Rub the oils, blended with either a carrier oil or a lotion, vigorously into the chilblains (but only unbroken ones). In the long term you should be looking at improving your circulation, either by massaging your feet or by using oils in the bath or in a foot bath. You could also use rosemary, lemon grass, ginger or marjoram for this purpose.

> **Caution**
> Anybody suffering from high blood pressure or epilepsy should avoid rosemary oil.

## HOMEOPATHIC REMEDIES

Tamus ointment is often soothing for chilblains.

- **Agaricus 6c**

For burning, itching and redness that is worse for cold.

- **Petroleum 6c**

For burning chilblains that itch, skin cracks.

- **Plantago 6c**

For skin that itches, burns and is sensitive.

**DOSAGE** 1 tablet three times daily. Maximum 2 weeks.

**LEFT** Ginger tea and rosemary oil can both help the circulation.

# Varicose veins

*Visible, often raised, unsightly and painful distended veins that commonly appear in the legs, although they can also occur in the walls of the rectum* (see Haemorrhoids on p.116); *they may ache after standing for long periods.*

Varicose veins occur when valves in the veins fail to work properly and impede the blood flow. There are often no symptoms, apart from their unsightly appearance. Although they are generally hereditary, they are frequently made worse by pregnancy, obesity, lack of exercise, jobs that involve prolonged standing, a sedentary lifestyle and by constipation. If they become chronic, the skin condition of varicose eczema may develop, and poor blood supply to the skin may result in severe ulcers from the most minor knocks and bumps.

## Call the doctor

*If the skin starts to ulcerate over or near a varicose vein.*

### CONVENTIONAL MEDICINE

For varicose veins in the legs, a well-fitting supportive elastic stocking that includes a heel, worn all day, may improve the symptoms. Surgical treatment may relieve them, although they may recur.

### HOMEOPATHIC REMEDIES

**Hamamelis 6c**
For varicose veins that feel bruised and sore. Veins large, blue. Varicose veins in pregnancy.

**Pulsatilla 6c**
For legs that feel heavy. Varicose veins itchy in warmth.

**Fluoricum acidum 6c**
For painful varicose veins. Varicose ulcers that have red edges.

**Ferrum metallicum 6c**
For varicose veins during pregnancy.

**DOSAGE** 1 tablet twice daily until improved, or for 10 days. May be repeated.

### HERBAL REMEDIES

Herbs like buckwheat, which is rich in rutin, can be used to strengthen the veins, while melilot, horse chestnut, motherwort, prickly ash or yarrow can be used to improve the circulation, combat any tendency to thrombosis and counter the deposit of fibrin that can cause further damage.

**USE AND DOSAGE** These herbs can be taken in teas or tinctures (try equal amounts of melilot, motherwort or yarrow, for example).

Externally, distilled witch hazel or horse chestnut ointment can be used in gentle massage.

### AROMATHERAPY

~ Cypress *(Cupressus sempervirens)*
~ Geranium *(Pelargonium graveolens)*

These oils are stimulating and also help to increase the circulation.

**APPLICATION** Put the essential oils into a carrier oil or lotion that can be massaged above the varicose veins – never over or below the veins. A warm compress can be placed on the vein if it is very painful and throbbing. Putting your legs higher than your head for at least 10 minutes twice a day will also help. Avoid constipation (see p.96), as this simply puts even more pressure on the veins.

### NUTRITION

If you already have varicose veins, your nutrition should be improved to provide an abundance of nutrients that are beneficial to the circulation. Eat buckwheat – as pancakes, or added to bread or biscuit recipes, for its rutin, a bioflavonoid that specifically strengthens blood vessels. Also eat plenty of avocados, olive oil and all the nuts and seeds for their vitamin E; liver, sardines, eggs, shellfish and pumpkin seeds for their zinc; and citrus fruit, blackcurrants, blackberries, blueberries, bilberries and dark red cherries for bioflavonoids and vitamin C.

Excessive amounts of caffeine and alcohol have an adverse effect on the heart and blood vessels, thus reducing the efficiency of the circulatory system. A high salt intake encourages fluid retention, swelling and high blood pressure, while refined carbohydrates and too much sugar lead to constipation and weight gain.

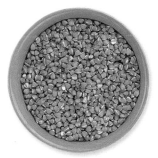

**ABOVE** Buckwheat is a herb that can be used to strengthen the veins.

### Prevention
*The major preventative step is to avoid constipation (see p.96) – plenty of fluid and the right kind of fibre are the key. And make lifestyle changes to control your weight.*

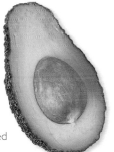

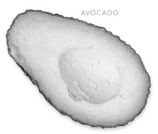

AVOCADO

# Restless legs

PASSION FLOWER

*Typified by a burning feeling, weakness or numbness, or by jerky movements in the legs, commonly occurring in women either just before going to sleep or soon after they sit down.*

**S**ymptoms of this usually minor, but nonetheless unpleasant, problem start as soon as you sit down or go to bed. Restless legs may be caused by prescribed drugs or by a problem in the central nervous system, but both these situations are rare; more often they are a symptom of iron-deficiency anaemia or are caused by circulation problems, but sometimes the complaint occurs for no apparent reason.

## 🌐 Call the doctor

*If you suddenly start suffering from this problem and the condition is severe and intractable.*

**BELOW** Boosting your iron intake might calm jerky legs that keep you awake at night.

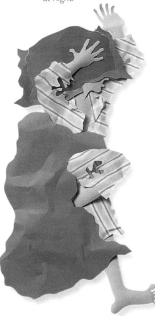

## ✚ CONVENTIONAL MEDICINE

Restless legs may occasionally be due to an iron deficiency, which can easily be treated by means of iron supplements.

## ✿ HOMEOPATHIC REMEDIES

🍃 **Zincum 6c**
For twitching, constant movement of feet both night and day.

🍃 **Tarantula 6c**
For restless feet and legs in bed, with weakness and numbness. Restless sleep. Legs restless in evening and before going to bed.

**DOSAGE** I tablet three times daily. Maximum 2 weeks or until improved.

## ▱ HERBAL REMEDIES

Teas to soothe and relax the nerves are worth trying, especially camomile, lemon balm, skullcap, vervain and passionflower. If the problem is particularly severe at night, it is worth bathing the legs in cramp-bark decoction or massaging a little cream containing the herb into the legs before going to bed.

**USE AND DOSAGE** I–2 drops of camomile, rose or lavender oil in 5ml/1tsp of almond oil also makes a good massage.

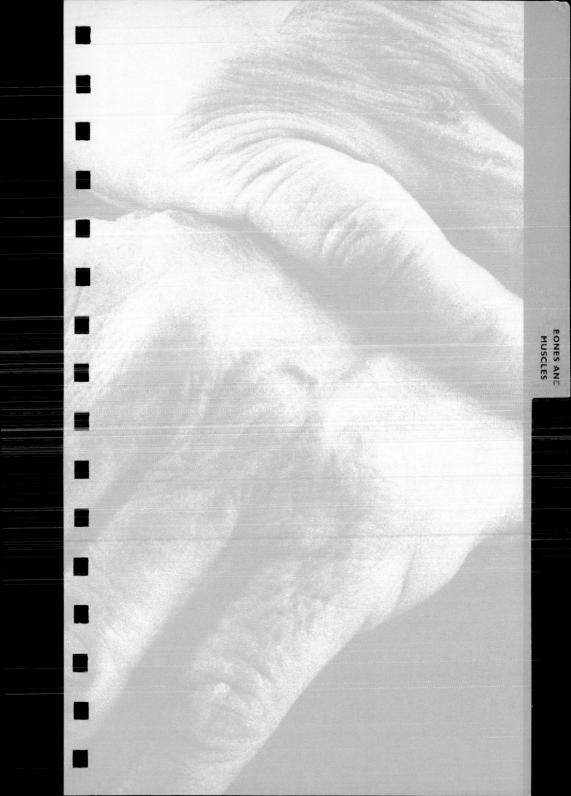

BONES AND
MUSCLES

# Bones and Muscles

The human skeleton contains more than 200 bones, which are moved by muscles and connected by ligaments and joints, giving us our complex body framework. Injuries, strains, wear and tear and internal ill-health can all affect this support system, causing aches and pains as well as more serious conditions. Today disorders of the musculoskeletal system make up 25 per cent of all visits to the doctor. This section looks at how such ailments – back pain or arthritis, osteo-porosis or RSI – can be treated at home, so that we function at our optimum level.

# Back pain

*Pain may come on suddenly or be more long-standing; often worse after sitting or standing for long periods; may affect any part of the spine; low back pain may be associated with pain down the leg.*

**Y**ou have an almost **90 per cent chance of suffering from back pain at some time in your life, and are then twice as likely to suffer again. Most back pain can be relieved by manipulative therapy within the first 6 weeks, though in some cases surgery may be the only answer. Prevention is the best treatment; if you are already a sufferer, try to maintain your back in a strong, healthy and mobile state. Do not stay in bed for more than 48 hours, even with a severe attack – seek professional help as soon as possible.**

## 🌐 Call the doctor

*If you cannot control when you pass urine or open your bowels; if you have numbness in a limb or difficulty moving it; if you have pain passing down your leg; if you cannot control the pain; if there is no improvement after 4–6 weeks.*

### Caution

*Make sure that back pain is properly diagnosed. Always read pain-reliever packages carefully, and do not exceed the stated dose.*

### ✚ CONVENTIONAL MEDICINE

Take a pain reliever regularly. This may need to be combined with a prescribed muscle relaxant. Try to avoid prolonged bed rest. If problems persist for more than a few days, early referral to a physiotherapist is recommended.

DOSAGE: ADULTS 1–2 tablets of pain relievers at onset of pain, repeated every 4 hours; consult pack.
DOSAGE: CHILDREN Give regular doses of liquid pain reliever; consult pack, or follow medical advice.

### HERBAL REMEDIES

Herbal remedies can ease symptoms, but where back pain is related to a mechanical fault, like a slipped disc, manipulative treatment is preferable.
USE AND DOSAGE Low back pain may be associated with kidney problems, so remedies like buchu, corn silk and couchgrass (2tsp of each per cup of tea) can help.

To ease local discomfort, soak a compress in 100ml/3½fl oz of hot water containing cramp bark (15ml/1tbsp) and cinnamon (5 ml/1tsp) tinctures, then apply. Reheat the mix and reapply as required. Anti-inflammatories such as devil's claw (6 × 200mg capsules daily) can also help.

## NUTRITION

Eat plenty of celery and parsley to encourage fluid elimination; turnips for their anti-inflammatory action; pineapple for its pain-relieving enzymes; and oily fish to maintain mobility. Reduce your intake of caffeine. Avoid carrying excessive weight, which puts even more strain on the spine.

## HOMEOPATHIC REMEDIES

Numbness in the bottom, or difficulty in knowing when you want to pass urine or open the bowels, requires urgent medical assessment.

**Bryonia 6c**

For stiffness in small of back at change of weather. Slow onset, worse for movement. Better for pressure, rest and cold applications.

**Gnaphalium 6c**

For pain extending down the leg, 'sciatica' with numbness. Worse on right side, for lying down and motion. Better for sitting in chair, drawing legs up.

**Tellurium 6c**

For pain extending down the leg, sciatica, right-sided. Pain worse for cough, sneezing, opening the bowels or touch. Also lumbago.

DOSAGE 1 tablet every 2–4 hours, for up to 3–4 days.

## AROMATHERAPY

It is important to have a good diagnosis.

FOR MUSCULAR PROBLEMS

**Lavender** (*Lavandula angustifolia*)

**Ginger** (*Zingiber officinale*)

**Marjoram** (*Origanum majorana*)

FOR KIDNEY PAIN AND DISC PROBLEMS

**Lavender** (*Lavandula angustifolia*)

**Roman camomile** (*Chamaemelum nobile*)

**Marjoram** (*Origanum majorana*) [for disc problems only]

The oils for muscular problems are warming and soothing; those for kidney pain and disc problems are soothing and help to kill the pain.

APPLICATION Use the oils for muscular pain in a massage; and all oils in the bath or in a compress.

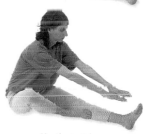

LEFT This exercise will stretch the hamstring and ease back pain. Sit on the floor with one leg straight and the other knee bent, with the foot flat on the floor.

LEFT Allow the raised knee to fall to the side.

ABOVE Gently stretch your arms forwards. Relax, then stretch again in a gentle rhythm for about 20 seconds. Repeat on the other side.

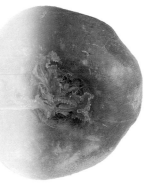

BELOW Eat turnips as a natural alternative to prescribed anti-inflammatory drugs.

# Arthritis

*Aching, stiff joints, commonly in the fingers, wrists, elbows, shoulders, knees, ankles and feet; joints are often swollen and may also be an abnormal shape; symptoms may be minor or cause considerable pain.*

There are more than 200 forms of arthritis that cause problems with the joints. Pain, stiffness, swelling and inflammation are generally present, but conditions may range from the inconvenience of arthritis in a finger, caused by an injury 20 years before, to severe disablement from rheumatoid arthritis. Some of the more serious conditions do not lend themselves to home remedies, but whatever form of arthritis you have, diet can play a key role in reducing its severity. Osteoarthritis and rheumatoid arthritis also respond to self-help, though this is not a substitute for surgery or drug therapy.

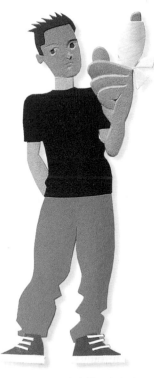

**ABOVE** Arthritis pain in the joints can be alleviated in part by changes in diet.

### CONVENTIONAL MEDICINE

Relieve arthritis with simple pain relievers such as paracetamol or aspirin. Sore joints may feel better when supported with a firm bandage. Keeping your joints warm may help, too, while gentle exercise is important to keep them supple.

DOSAGE: ADULTS 1–2 tablets of pain relievers at onset of pain, repeated every 4 hours; consult pack for details.

DOSAGE: CHILDREN Give regular doses of liquid pain reliever; consult pack, or follow medical advice.

### HERBAL REMEDIES

Anti-inflammatory herbs, such as birch, black cohosh, meadowsweet, poplar and willow, are widely used – usually as teas, although birch sap (collected in the autumn and taken in teaspoon doses) was once a popular folk remedy. Devil's claw root, from the Kalahari, is now popular.

USE AND DOSAGE Take up to 3g of devil's claw root powder daily in capsules, for at least 4 weeks.

Combine 10 drops of rosemary or wintergreen oil with 5ml/1tsp of infused comfrey oil, then use as a gentle massage.

## HOMEOPATHIC REMEDIES

It is helpful to consult a qualified homeopath.

**Bryonia 6c**

For joints that are red, hot, with tearing pains. Worse for slightest movement. Better for holding joint tightly, applying heat. Dry mouth and thirst.

**Rhododendrum 6c**

For arthritis that affects smaller joints, which feel weak. Worse for changes of weather, and before storms and cold winters. Better for warmth.

DOSAGE 1 tablet three times daily. Maximum 1 month.

## AROMATHERAPY

- Lavender *(Lavandula angustifolia)*
- Roman camomile *(Chamaemelum nobile)*
- Eucalyptus *(Eucalyptus radiata)*
- Juniper *(Juniperus communis)*
- Ginger *(Zingiber officinale)*

These oils have a painkilling effect, especially for localized pain. They are also warming and soothing. But there are many oils that can be used: experiment to find out which ones suit you best.

APPLICATION Use in foot or hand baths, depending on where the affected joints are, or massage an oil or lotion into the body. If your joint problem is recent, check your stress levels are as low as possible.

## NUTRITION

Drink ginger tea and make sure that you add plenty of fresh ginger root and dried ginger to recipes. Include parsley, celery and watercress in your diet.

For all arthritic conditions, except gout, eat plenty of oily fish and shellfish, for their omega-3 fatty acids; sweet potatoes, broccoli, apricots, carrots and liver for their vitamin A and beta-carotene; citrus fruit, strawberries, kiwis and dark green vegetables for their vitamin C and bioflavonoids; olive oil, sunflower seeds, unsalted nuts and avocados for their vitamin E. Reduce your intake of red meat, coffee and game. Gout sufferers must avoid all alcohol, game, offal, yeast and meat extracts, all oily fish, fish roe, mussels and scallops.

### Prevention

*Being seriously overweight adds greatly to the stresses on all weight-bearing joints and will predispose you to arthritis in the lower spine, hips, knees, ankles and feet.*

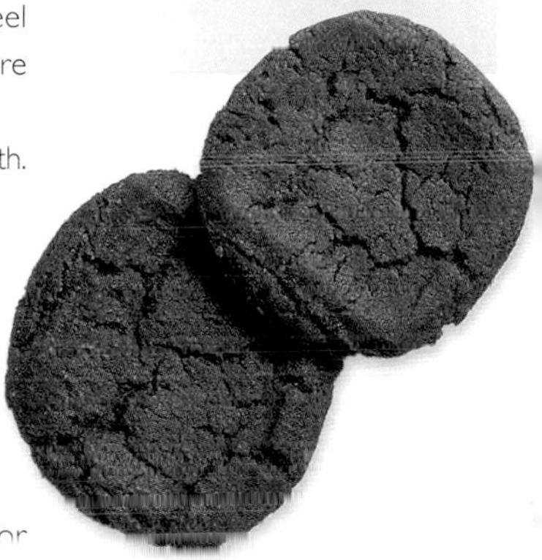

ABOVE Introduce ginger into your diet, as well as drinking ginger tea and using in oil for massage.

### Caution

*If you are using a compress, or a warm hand or foot bath (or just a warm bath), make sure that you mobilize the joints as much as possible afterwards, because the heat can cause congestion, making matters worse.*

# Osteoarthritis

*Stiff, painful joints, which often become hard and swollen as
the cartilage between the bones, which acts as a cushion,
wears away; may affect any joint, but is common in the hips,
knees, spine and fingers.*

steoarthritis is commonly seen as the result of long-term wear
and tear on weight-bearing joints, often as the result of occupa-
tion or sporting activities. However, this is not the only cause, and previous injury or fracture, damage to the cartilage (especially in the knee),
previous infection, congenital deformity (such as spinal curvature) or
bunions may also lead to osteoarthritis.

## Prevention

*Maintaining a sensible weight
and avoiding activities likely to
lead to stress-related arthritis
are the key factors. Marathon
running, relentless jogging and
high-impact aerobics can all
damage joint surfaces.*

## CONVENTIONAL MEDICINE

Try to stay as active as possible, which helps to
keep the affected joints supple, increase muscle
strength and control weight gain, which can aggravate osteoarthritis. Staying active may mean taking
pain relievers and using mechanical aids, such as a
walking frame or stick. Your doctor can arrange for
physiotherapy, if required. In severe cases, a joint
replacement can provide a new lease of life.

**DOSAGE: ADULTS** 1–2 tablets of pain reliever at
onset of pain, repeated every 4 hours; consult pack.

**BELOW** Peppers and nuts
can help to protect joints.

## NUTRITION

Oily fish are an important food group: the omega-3
fatty acids they contain are naturally anti-inflammatory and help to maintain joint mobility. Eat plenty
of liver, carrots, sweet potatoes, spinach, broccoli, apricots, mangoes and cantaloupe melons
for their vitamin A and beta-carotene, which
are equally important nutrients; all the green
leafy vegetables, citrus fruit, kiwis, red, yellow
and green peppers for their vitamin C, which
helps to protect the joints from further damage.
Avoid red meat and meat products as far as
possible – instead, use fish, poultry, nuts, seeds and
beans, together with eggs and modest amounts of
low-fat dairy products, as protein sources.

Ginger tea can be soothing. Peel and grate 1cm/ ½in of fresh ginger root, add to a mug of boiling water, cover and steep for 10 minutes. Strain and add 1 tsp of honey; drink two or three mugs a day.

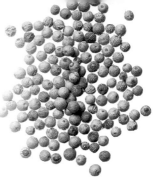

**ABOVE** Black pepper oil makes an effective massage or bath oil for osteoarthritis.

### HERBAL REMEDIES

A number of herbs may help this condition.

USE AND DOSAGE The 'wear and tear' contributing to osteoarthritis may be eased by regular use of comfrey cream or infused oil: massage a little into the aching joint every night for at least 2 months.

Internally, herbs to stimulate circulation and clear toxins can help – try a decoction of angelica, yellow dock, prickly ash and willow bark (1–2tsp per cup).

Devil's claw root is useful (see *Arthritis* on p.66).

### HOMEOPATHIC REMEDIES

A consultation with a homeopath is recommended.

~ **Rhus toxicodendron 6c**

For tearing pains, worse at night, restless with them. Pain worse for initial movement, then improves as gets moving. Joints feel sore and stiff. Worse for wet or cold weather.

~ **Pulsatilla 6c**

For pains that are wandering from joint to joint. Weepy with the pains and emotional. Pains better for gentle motion. Worse for warmth.

DOSAGE 1 tablet three times daily. Maximum 2 weeks.

### AROMATHERAPY

~ Lavender *(Lavandula angustifolia)*
~ Roman camomile *(Chamaemelum nobile)*
~ Marjoram *(Origanum majorana)*
~ Ginger *(Zingiber officinale)*
~ Black pepper *(Piper nigrum)*
~ Rosemary *(Rosmarinus officinalis)*
~ Juniper *(Juniperus communis)*

These oils are warming and soothing. Juniper also helps detoxify the system.

APPLICATION Use in warm baths, in hand or foot baths. You can also add them to massage oils or lotions, but do not massage over any inflamed area.

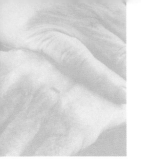

# Osteoporosis

*Characterized by a weakening of the bones, but does not cause any actual symptoms, although it is the commonest cause of fractures in people over the age of 75; carries a strong familial link.*

steoporosis – the condition in which the bones become weak, brittle and easily broken – normally occurs in women after the menopause, though men can get it, too. It is growing at an alarming rate and must be seen as an extremely serious problem. Any medical condition that causes a premature menopause *(see p.110)* increases the risk of osteoporosis; this is also true of long-term treatment with some drugs and of eating disorders like anorexia and bulimia. Diseases that affect the body's absorption of nutrients – particularly Crohn's disease, colitis and diverticulitis – also predispose you to a greater risk.

**BELOW** Weight-bearing exercise is fundamental to the treatment of osteoporosis.

## CONVENTIONAL MEDICINE

To avoid the risk of osteoporosis, encourage children to take regular weight-bearing exercise and to drink plenty of milk. Calcium and vitamin D supplements are also recommended in older women, either through the diet or prescribed tablets. Avoid smoking and excessive alcohol consumption. HRT prevents osteoporosis and can be taken at any stage after the menopause, usually for at least 5 years. If osteoporosis is already present, it can be treated with prescribed drugs. Try to continue taking exercise to improve muscle tone and bulk.

## HOMEOPATHIC REMEDIES

In homeopathy the patient is treated according to the symptoms that the body produces. As a disease, osteoporosis does not have symptoms until a fracture occurs, so there are no specific remedies.

## NUTRITION

The key to avoiding osteoporosis is building strong bones from the teens onwards, but sadly this is also the time when many girls get on the dieting treadmill. Having a low calcium intake in the early years is almost a guarantee of having problem bones later on. The average woman who is modestly active needs around 2,000 calories per day; it is impossible to get all the nutrients you need to build strong bones on very low-calorie diets (under 1,250 calories per day).

The diet of all women should be rich in foods that contain calcium, vitamin D, bioflavonoids, vitamin K and magnesium. For calcium, eat plenty of low-fat dairy products, nuts, beans and tinned sardines (with their bones); for vitamin D, eat eggs and oily fish; for vitamin C and bioflavonoids eat citrus fruit (with some of the pith and skin), blackcurrants, bilberries, blueberries and blackberries; for vitamin K, eat spinach, broccoli and cabbage; eat tofu, almonds and cashews for their magnesium

BLACKBERRIES

**ABOVE** Vitamin D, found in oily fish, is needed for the absorption of calcium.

### Caution

*Do not use rosemary or fennel oil if you have high blood pressure or epilepsy.*

### AROMATHERAPY

- Fennel *(Foeniculum vulgare)*
- Rosemary *(Rosmarinus officinalis)*
- Black pepper *(Piper nigrum)*
- Lavender *(Lavandula angustifolia)*
- Roman camomile *(Chamaemelum nobile)*
- Marjoram *(Origanum majorana)*
- Benzoin *(Styrax benzoin)*

These oils are warming, soothing and anti inflammatory. Fennel contains plant oestrogens

**APPLICATION** Use in baths, foot baths or bowls of warm water. They can also be massaged in.

### HERBAL REMEDIES

Herbs rich in minerals, vitamins and steroidal compounds are recommended to combat bone loss in old age and can contribute greatly to dietary needs. **USE AND DOSAGE** Drink a daily tea of stinging nettles, alfalfa and sage (2tsp per cup) and take 10ml/2tsp of horsetail juice in water three times daily.

Chinese angelica (Dang Gui) also provides nourishment and is becoming more available in tablets from health-food stores.

ROMAN CAMOMILE

# Rheumatism

*Characterized by general aches and pains that affect the muscles, tendons and connective tissue – often, but not always, surrounding the joints; may be accompanied by stiffness.*

**R**heumatism is a vague and general term describing aching joints or muscles, but it is not a specific disease. **RSI** *(see p.76)*, tennis elbow, frozen shoulder and tendonitis are just some of the disorders that can be grouped together under the broad heading of rheumatism. Even fibrositis is part of this collection. None of them is linked to osteoarthritis or rheumatoid arthritis. Your doctor may offer you anti-inflammatory drugs or even steroid injections, but there are home remedies that may be just as effective. Unless you are in severe pain, try these first, as none of them has any side-effects.

## 🌐 Call the doctor

*If your symptoms persist for a period of longer than 3–4 weeks.*

### Caution

*Do not use rosemary oil if you suffer from high blood pressure or epilepsy.*

### ✚ CONVENTIONAL MEDICINE

Often resting for a few days, followed by gentle stretching exercises, is all that is required. A warm hot-water bottle or ice pack can help. Some people find that a firm supportive bandage provides enormous relief. Take pain relievers as required. Your doctor may want to arrange for further investigations if the symptoms persist.

**DOSAGE: ADULTS** 1–2 tablets of pain reliever at onset of pain, repeated every 4 hours; consult pack.

**DOSAGE: CHILDREN** Give regular doses of liquid pain reliever; consult pack, or follow medical advice.

### AROMATHERAPY

- Lavender *(Lavandula angustifolia)*
- Roman camomile *(Chamaemelum nobile)*
- Juniper *(Juniperus communis)*
- Marjoram *(Origanum majorana)*
- Ginger *(Zingiber officinale)*
- Benzoin *(Styrax benzoin)*
- Rosemary *(Rosmarinus officinalis)*

Some of these oils may be more beneficial to you than others, so experiment for yourself.

**APPLICATION** Use in the bath (except benzoin), or

in a compress over the affected area. You can also use them in a massage medium: never massage over swollen and inflamed joints; massage instead over the affected area between flare-ups.

### HERBAL REMEDIES

Anti-inflammatory rubs (such as 5 drops of camomile essence in 5ml/1tsp of infused St John's wort oil) can be helpful for tennis elbow or frozen shoulder. Rheumatism may respond to cleansing teas, which remove toxins in the tissues.

USE AND DOSAGE Try an infusion of bogbean, meadowsweet and yarrow leaves (2tsp), flavoured with a little lemon juice.

Warm compresses may help: soak a cloth in cramp-bark and angelica decoction.

**RIGHT** Step forward with one foot, keeping your hands high. Hold, then repeat on the other side.

### HOMEOPATHIC REMEDIES

If the following do not help, consult a homeopath.

🐌 Colchicum 6c

For severe inflammation of joints, with severe pain. Person is irritable. Worse for any motion. May affect several joints at once, or move from left to right side. Worse at night. Also used for gout.

🐌 Dulcamara 6c

For stiff and painful joints. Worse in autumn, for cold and damp, getting wet. Better for moving, dry weather. May also have diarrhoea.

DOSAGE 1 tablet three times daily. Maximum 2 weeks.

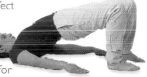

**ABOVE** This position will improve hip and knee flexibility and strengthen the back.

### NUTRITION

Eat plenty of oily fish and all the powerful antioxidant foods, which are rich in vitamins A, C and E (see *Arthritis* on p.66) and in the minerals zinc and selenium. Use celery seeds (not celery salt) liberally in cooking. Avoid foods that will aggravate your inflammation, like red meat; and those likely to increase your levels of uric acid, such as offal, yeast, yeast extracts, meat extracts, roe and even caviar; avoid all red and fortified wines, and drink modestly other forms of alcohol. Do not drink more than 1–2 cups of coffee a day.

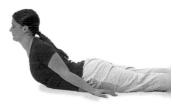

**ABOVE** Raising the chest while keeping the hips on the floor preserves mobility and strength in the spine.

# Cramp

*Sudden and continuous pain in a muscle, often the calf or foot, although it can flare up anywhere in the body; the pain, caused by involuntary contraction of the muscle, may develop during exercise or at night.*

This sudden condition always seems to strike at the most inappropriate moments. It is most common in the calf muscles and is excruciatingly uncomfortable, often leaving you feeling as though you have been kicked by a mule. The common wisdom is that it is due to a deficiency of salt, but this is hardly ever the case. Potassium deficiency is a far more likely cause. Cramp can also occur if the muscles are not receiving enough oxygen because the blood supply is damaged. Cramps at night are common in pregnant women and the elderly, although they may be a sign of a more serious underlying condition, such as diabetes.

## Call the doctor

*If you have experienced pain in the chest or calves during exercise.*

## Prevention

*Occupational cramps are caused by relentless but controlled repetitive movements. Practise some relaxation techniques and take regular breaks.*

### CONVENTIONAL MEDICINE

Cramp-like pain will usually go away when the muscle is relaxed. This generally means resting for a few minutes. Cramps at night are often relieved by stretching and rubbing the affected muscle. Pain in the chest or calves during exercise, which stops after resting, can be more serious and may require medical attention.

### NUTRITION

Nutrition is often the key to relieving attacks of cramp, but it must be seen as a long-term benefit, and not as an instant cure. If you suffer regularly from cramp, eat at least one banana each day for the potassium that it contains. Vitamin E is a great aid to the circulation, so eat avocados, nuts, seeds and lots of good olive oil. Sardines contain beneficial omega-3 fatty acids and also are a rich source of calcium, as are all dairy products. Eat natural yogurt for its riboflavin, and eggs for their vitamin $B_{12}$. A glass of Indian tonic water taken at bedtime – without the gin – often helps, due to its quinine content.

To help alleviate or prevent cramp take 400 IU of vitamin E each day and a good mineral supplement containing calcium, potassium and magnesium.

## HOMEOPATHIC REMEDIES

**Cuprum metallicum 6c**
For violent, sudden cramps in the calves at night. Useful for cramps that occur during pregnancy. Try this remedy first.

**Magnesium phosphoricum 6c**
For writer's cramp, cramps from prolonged exertion. Cramps in the calves better for rubbing.

**Nux vomica 6c**
For cramps in the calves and soles, with lots of muscle spasms. Sleeplessness, particularly towards morning, with dreams of arguments. Person may be irritable.

DOSAGE I tablet before retiring. Maximum 2 weeks

## HERBAL REMEDIES

Decoctions of cramp bark or black haw can help persistent night cramp, while teas of wild yam, camomile or fennel can ease stomach cramps.

USE AND DOSAGE Add 1tsp of cramp bark or black haw to 1½ cups of water and simmer for 10 minutes to make a decoction.

Make an external rub using 5 drops each of cypress, marjoram and basil oils in 15ml/3tsp of almond oil.

## AROMATHERAPY

**Geranium** (Pelargonium gravcolens)
**Ginger** (Zingiber officinale)
**Cypress** (Cupressus sempervirens)
These oils are stimulating and increase the circulation, warming up the muscles so that cramp does not set in.

APPLICATION Use in a compress, in the bath or in a foot spa. You really need to be looking at prevention, rather than cure, so make sure that you massage the feet and legs in the evenings, before you go to bed, if you are susceptible to cramp.

**BELOW** Cypress oil heps to ease the pain caused by cramp.

MEADOWSWEET

# Repetitive strain injury: RSI

*Pain in the hand, wrist, forearm, shoulder and/or neck, often related to using a keyboard for long periods, although any repetitive task may bring it on.*

Repetitive strain injury is a result of overuse of the upper body at work, but should properly be called work-related upper-limb injury. The best treatment may be rest and home remedies.

## CONVENTIONAL MEDICINE

Ensure that your keyboard, monitor and desk are comfortable and ergonomically safe. Take a break at regular intervals and rest until any pain has gone completely. If it persists, try a non-steroidal anti-inflammatory pain reliever. Your doctor may suggest that you see a specialist.

DOSAGE: ADULTS 1–2 tablets of pain reliever at onset of pain, repeated every 4 hours; consult pack.

## HERBAL REMEDIES

Anti-inflammatory herbs like meadowsweet, white willow or St John's wort may be helpful in teas.

USE AND DOSAGE Use 2tsp of these herbs per cup. Herbal rubs for rheumatism *(see p.72)* and arthritis *(see p.66)* may provide relief.

Siberian ginseng, astragalus or shiitake mushrooms may improve some chronic conditions.

## HOMEOPATHIC REMEDIES

### Arnica 6c

For bruised sensation in muscles and tendons. Aching muscles after overexertion. Worse for damp weather and continuing movement. Person says they are fine, even when obviously not.

### Causticum 6c

For burning pain, inflamed tendons. Pain worse for draughts, cold or overuse. Carpal tunnel syndrome. Person is very idealistic and intense.

DOSAGE 1 tablet twice daily. Maximum 2 weeks.

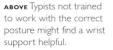

**ABOVE** Typists not trained to work with the correct posture might find a wrist support helpful.

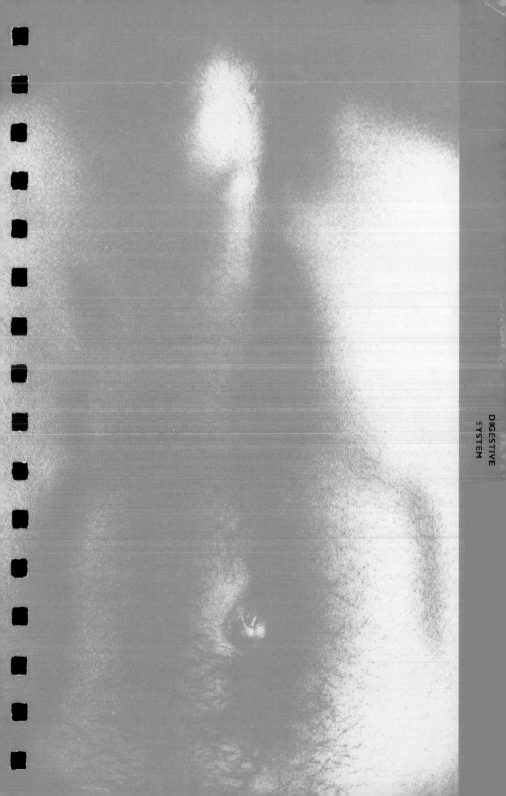

DIGESTIVE
SYSTEM

# The Digestive System

**D**igestion enables the body to convert the food that we eat into energy and use it to build and repair tissues. A healthy digestive system is vital for general well-being, but in our rushed modern lifestyles it is often abused, leading to many of the problems that plague our daily lives, from indigestion and abdominal pain to peptic ulcers and gastroenteritis. Weight concerns – either too much or too little – are another manifestation of digestive problems. But with a little thought and a sensible diet, many of these ailments can be treated.

# Heartburn

*Burning sensation in upper abdomen, going up the centre of the chest to the back of the throat, often with an acid taste in the mouth; pain may be worse at night, when lying flat, bending or stooping.*

**H**eartburn, also known as acid indigestion, may be caused by obesity, the late stages of pregnancy or a hiatus hernia, but most often results from too much of the wrong kind of food or plain overeating. The acid contents of the stomach escape upwards into the oesophagus, causing the characteristic burning sensation behind the breastbone. Whatever the cause, home remedies can help resolve the discomfort.

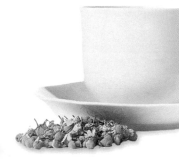

**ABOVE** Herbal teas containing caraway, cardamom, ginger or tangerine can help relieve heartburn.

### 🌐 Call the doctor

*If heartburn continues for a long period of time, as it can be indicative of complaints such as ulcers or gallstones; if the symptoms persist or are not relieved by an antacid.*

### ✚ CONVENTIONAL MEDICINE

Avoid eating fatty foods or consuming hot drinks or alcohol. Try to stop smoking and lose weight if necessary. If the symptoms are worse at night, drink a glass of milk before bedtime and raise the head of the bed. Take an antacid if the symptoms continue.

DOSAGE: ADULTS AND CHILDREN OVER 16 Many types of antacid are available in tablet or liquid form. Be aware that they contain magnesium or aluminium salts, or both: the former (e.g. Milk of Magnesia) tend to cause diarrhoea; the latter (e.g. Aluminium hydroxide) constipation. Some antacids are combined with alginic acid and are particularly helpful for heartburn; consult pack for details.

### HERBAL REMEDIES

Soothing, demulcent herbs, such as marsh-mallow and slippery elm, are widely used for heartburn.

USE AND DOSAGE Take these herbs in tablets or capsules (200mg) before meals.

Teas of antacid herbs, such as meadowsweet, centaury, bogbean, dandelion or black horehound, can also be useful.

Carminative teas used for indigestion (see p.80) may help, or make a thin gruel by mixing 1 tsp of powdered slippery-elm bark with a little water, then add a hot camomile infusion. Drink before meals.

### ❖ HOMEOPATHIC REMEDIES

Persistent heartburn requires medical assessment, but a consultation with a homeopath may help.

🐌 **Robina 6c**

For heartburn with acidity. Worse at night and for lying down. Prevents sleep. Abdomen bloated with wind and colic. Headaches.

🐌 **Sulphur 6c**

For heartburn from eating either too much, or spicy, food. Big appetite, craves spices, alcohol, fats. Thirsty for cold drinks.

**DOSAGE** 1 tablet hourly for six doses. May be repeated if necessary.

### 🍎 NUTRITION

Avoiding the symptoms of heartburn is simply a matter of applying common sense to your eating habits. Avoid alcohol, nicotine and caffeine. Do not overeat or eat very acidic or irritant foods, such as chilli, pickles, raw onion, sour fruit and very hot curries, or deep-fried foods. If you have a hiatus hernia or are in the later stages of pregnancy, make sure that you eat little and often, spreading your daily intake over five meals instead of three. Use all the good digestive herbs routinely – mint, dill, fennel, ginger and slippery elm (see *Gastritis* on p.104) – and end your meals with a glass of mint tea. Heartburn for which there is no obvious reason sometimes responds well to a few weeks on the food combining (Hay) diet (see p.200).

### 💧 AROMATHERAPY

🐌 Fennel *(Foeniculum vulgare)*

🐌 Peppermint *(Mentha piperita)*

🐌 Black pepper *(Piper nigrum)*

🐌 Roman camomile *(Chamaemelum nobile)*

🐌 Ginger *(Zingiber officinale)*

These oils both calm and soothe the digestive tract.

**APPLICATION** Use in a massage oil or lotion, or in a warm compress on the stomach area.

**Prevention**

*Obesity must be dealt with, because it is a major cause of heartburn. Simply losing weight and avoiding tight, restrictive clothes will make an enormous difference.*

**Caution**

*If you are pregnant, do not take any medicines without first consulting your doctor.*

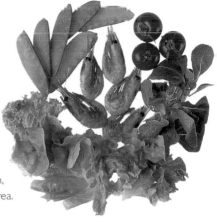

**BELOW** Sometimes heartburn can be eased by following the principles of food combining.

# Indigestion

*Pain or discomfort experienced in the upper part of the abdomen, related to food; it may be associated with nausea and burping; the tendency to indigestion often increases with age.*

**T**here cannot be a single person who has not had the occasional bout of indigestion and, with the exception of underlying diseases being the cause, it is always self-inflicted. Indigestion starts in a kitchen and that is where you will find the answer.

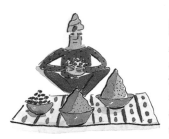

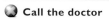

### 🌑 Call the doctor

*If you have a persistent problem with indigestion; if you have the symptoms and have lost weight unintentionally; it is the first time you have had these symptoms and you are over 40 years old.*

### ✚ CONVENTIONAL MEDICINE

Avoid eating immediately before bedtime, plus alcohol, cigarettes and tight-fitting clothes. Raising the head of the bed may help. When the pain starts, try drinking milk; if that does not help, take an antacid. If the symptoms do not respond, then a short course of cimetidine or ranitidine may help.

DOSAGE: ADULTS AND CHILDREN OVER 16  For information on antacids, *see Heartburn on p.78*. Other indigestion mixtures contain dimethicone to relieve wind; consult pack for details.

Take 200mg cimetidine, or 75mg ranitidine with water, when the symptoms appear; repeat after 1 hour if symptoms persist. Maximum daily cimetidine dose: 800mg, but not more than 400mg in any 4 hours. Maximum daily ranitidine dose: 300 mg. To prevent night-time heartburn take 100mg cimetidine 1 hour before bedtime. If symptoms continue after 2 weeks, seek medical advice. Avoid both cimetidine and ranitidine in pregnancy.

### ▱ HERBAL REMEDIES

Herbal carminatives like caraway, cardamom, ginger, galangal and dried tangerine peel/Chen Pi may help.
USE AND DOSAGE  Make a standard infusion or use these herbs in tinctures (2.5ml/½tsp diluted with water, or up to 20 drops on the tongue).

Slippery elm or marsh-mallow-root capsules will help protect the stomach lining.

## HOMEOPATHIC REMEDIES

Persistent symptoms require medical attention, but a consultation with a homeopath may be helpful.

#### Lycopodium 30c

For burning in throat. Pressure in stomach and bitter taste in mouth. Bloating immediately after meals. Craves warm drinks.

#### Nux vomica 30c

For pain, like a stone, in the stomach some time after meals, together with nausea. Indigestion from drinking strong coffee.

#### Carbo vegetabilis 30c

For heaviness, fullness, sleepiness after food. Food turns to gas in stomach, with belching and flatus.

DOSAGE 1 tablet hourly for six doses, then three times daily. Maximum 1 week.

ABOVE Ginger is an established treatment for nausea and indigestion.

## AROMATHERAPY

#### Fennel (Foeniculum vulgare)
#### Peppermint (Mentha x piperita)
#### Black pepper (Piper nigrum)
#### Roman camomile (Chamaemelum nobile)
#### Ginger (Zingiber officinale)

These oils calm and soothe the digestive tract.

APPLICATION Use in a massage oil or lotion, or in a warm compress over the stomach area.

## NUTRITION

RADISHES

Long gaps between meals, eating on the run, large, rich meals late at night and a surfeit of greasy or deep-fried food represent an assault on your digestive system. So eat a well-balanced diet with regular meals. Avoid eating too much of the obvious culprits – raw onions, pickles, hot, spicy chilli and curry, radishes, cucumber and peppers, unripe bananas are particularly indigestible. A glass of mint tea is an almost instant cure – specially sweetened with a bit of honey, one of the great digestive soothers. Another traditional remedy is a generous pinch of bicarbonate of soda dissolved on the tongue.

> ### Caution
> Severe pain after eating or when hungry, loss of blood in the stool and long-standing chronic digestive problems could be symptoms of a more serious condition. Avoid aspirin and NSAIDS, which may make the symptoms worse.

PEPPERMINT

# Nausea

*Sensation of impending vomiting, often accompanied by sweating, excessive salivation, dizziness and pale skin; in pregnancy it tends to be worst in the first 3–4 months, but may continue throughout in rare cases, at any time of day.*

Nausea, that familiar feeling of sickness, may be followed by vomiting. This violent expulsion of the stomach contents may bring relief if the vomiting has been triggered by overindulgence or the ingestion of some toxic substance. But it may also be the first of a series of repeated bouts in a prolonged episode, if the underlying cause is food poisoning or some other form of infection *(see Gastroenteritis on p.102)*. High temperatures in children, appendicitis, motion sickness, pregnancy, migraine, liver and gall-bladder disease, whooping cough, vertigo, Ménière's disease and severe anxiety can all cause nausea.

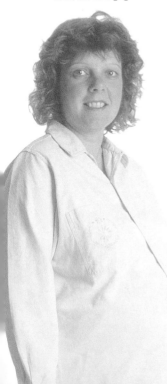

**BELOW** So-called morning sickness can happen at any time of day, but can be relieved by small amounts of food, such as a ginger biscuit.

### ✚ CONVENTIONAL MEDICINE

Avoid eating, but take frequent sips of plain water and lie down until the sensation passes. Anti-nausea treatments can be helpful, particularly for travel sickness, but consult your doctor, as the remedy may depend on the cause of the nausea. Nausea due to pregnancy may be relieved by eating: try eating frequent light snacks throughout the day, possibly even before getting up in the morning.

DOSAGE: ADULTS AND CHILDREN  Treatments for travel sickness are usually taken before travelling and then repeated at regular intervals; consult pack for details *(see also Motion Sickness on p.184)*.

### ▱ HERBAL REMEDIES

Ginger is probably the most widely used herb for nausea *(see p.184)*, but other useful remedies include camomile, peppermint, lemon balm and bitter orange.

USE AND DOSAGE  Take these herbs in teas or, more easily during bouts of nausea, as drops of tincture (diluted 50:50 with water) on the tongue.

Black horehound can be very effective, but its distinctive flavour makes some people feel worse.

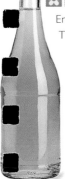

### ✿ HOMEOPATHIC REMEDIES

Ensure there is no serious medical condition.
These remedies are useful for morning sickness.

∞ **Ipecacuanha 6c**

For constant nausea, not relieved by vomiting.
Clean tongue, needs to keep swallowing an
excess of saliva.

∞ **Sepia 6c**

For nausea at sight, smell or thought of food.
Morning sickness before eating, vomits on
rinsing mouth. Craves vinegar.

∞ **Glossyplum 6c**

For nausea and vomiting worse before breakfast,
movement or standing up. No appetite, sensitive
stomach with a lot of gas.

**DOSAGE** 1 tablet every half-hour. Maximum 12 doses.

### ⬤ AROMATHERAPY

∞ Ginger *(Zingiber officinale)*
∞ Peppermint *(Mentha x piperita)*
∞ Lavender *(Lavandula angustifolia)*
∞ Roman camomile *(Chamaemelum nobile)*

Lavender and camomile are soothing and calming;
peppermint acts as a mild anaesthetic to the stomach wall; ginger is the universal remedy for nausea.
**APPLICATION** Use as a compress, and accompanied
by herbal teas.

### ⬤ NUTRITION

This depends on the cause of the nausea, but in
general terms a bout of food poisoning should
be treated with the BRAT diet *(see p.99)*,
followed by a gradual return to normal eating *(see Gastroenteritis on p.102)*. Vomiting
caused by ulcers needs a specific pattern of
eating *(see Gastritis on p.104)*. For nausea
caused by vertigo or Ménière's disease follow the advice for motion sickness *(see p.184)*.
The young and elderly can dehydrate rapidly as
a result of repeated vomiting – especially if
accompanied by diarrhoea. It is essential to replace
lost fluids *(see p.102)*.

> **Caution**
>
> *If you are pregnant,
> do not take any
> medicines without
> first consulting your
> doctor. If you have
> glaucoma, do not
> take medicines
> containing hyoscine.*

🔵 **Call the doctor**

*If nausea is a recurring
problem; if bouts of
nausea and vomiting have
no obvious explanation;
if you have been feeling
nauseous for more than
a week and you are
not pregnant.*

LAVENDER

# Abdominal pain

*Waves of cramping pain, often with diarrhoea and/or nausea – likely cause: gastroenteritis; severe, constant pain in lower right abdomen – likely cause: appendicitis; lower abdominal pain, with pain on passing urine – likely cause: cystitis.*

A bdominal pain (stomach ache) is the result of abusing your digestive system. Overindulgence, excessive alcohol, too much fat or unwise combinations of food may all be the culprit. It is a problem that most people will have occasionally; it can also be triggered by stress and anxiety. Regular attacks of stomach pain need investigation to rule out underlying disease. *(See also Constipation on p.96, Diarrhoea on p.98, Flatulence on p.86, Gall-Bladder Problems on p.88, Gastroenteritis on p.102, Irritable Bowel Syndrome on p.94, Peptic Ulcers on p.92).*

**BELOW** Many causes of abdominal pain can be attributed to some element of the diet.

## CONVENTIONAL MEDICINE

Stomach ache can initially be treated with a simple pain reliever, such as paracetamol (but not aspirin or ibuprofen). Drink plenty of water, and eat only if you are hungry. Avoid spicy or fatty foods until the pain subsides. If it becomes worse, or remains unchanged for several days, seek medical advice.

**DOSAGE: ADULTS** 1–2 tablets of pain relievers at onset of pain, repeated every 4 hours; consult pack for details.

**DOSAGE: CHILDREN** Give regular doses of liquid pain reliever; consult pack, or follow medical advice.

## HERBAL REMEDIES

Carminative herbs – aniseed, clove, coriander, fennel, ginger, parsley, peppermint and thyme – can help relieve the pain associated with wind. Bogbean, centaury, Irish moss and meadowsweet can ease the inflammation associated with overindulgence. If stress and anxiety are to blame, try regular cups of lemon balm or camomile infusion.

**USE AND DOSAGE** Use the herbs in standard infusions and decoctions; drink a cup every 3–4 hours while symptoms persist. Avoid laxative herbs if the cause of pain is uncertain.

### ❖ HOMEOPATHIC REMEDIES

These remedies may also be used for infantile colic.

**Magnesium phosphoricum 6c**

For cramping abdominal pains. Better for heat, pulling legs up to abdomen, pressure and rubbing. Belching gives no relief.

**Dioscorea 6c**

For colic pains. Better for stretching or for bending backwards.

**Colocynthis 6c**

For cutting colic pains. Better for pressure, heat. Pains after anger. Bends over double; presses on abdomen for relief.

**Chamomilla 6c**

For infant colic. Greenish stool, infant's cry is angry, pains are unbearable. Better for being carried.

**DOSAGE** 1 tablet every half-hour. Maximum six doses.

### AROMATHERAPY

**Lavender (*Lavandula angustifolia*)**
**Roman camomile (*Chamaemelum nobile*)**
Both oils are soothing and help to kill the pain.

**APPLICATION** Place a warm compress on the stomach and possibly on the lower back. A hot-water bottle can be used on top of the compress. If the pain continues and the reason is unknown, then good diagnosis is important. If the pain is due to constipation, gentle circular massage of the abdomen with lavender and camomile will help.

### NUTRITION

Everyone knows the proverb 'You are what you eat', and this is true in relation to all digestive problems. Eat plenty of foods containing soluble fibre, such as oats, apples, pears, root vegetables and all the bean family. When cooking vegetables, add a few caraway seeds; chew a few dill seeds and drink mint tea after meals. Reduce your intake of alcohol, coffee and all fizzy drinks. Eat little and often and cut down on all animal fats. A few weeks on the food combining (Hay) diet *(see p.200)* often works wonders for chronic digestive difficulties.

**Caution**

*Avoid taking aspirin or ibuprofen, as they may irritate an already sore stomach lining. If using essential oils on small children, make sure that the doses are the relevant sizes.*

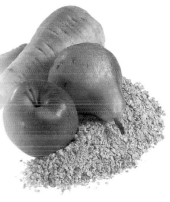

**ABOVE** Plenty of soluble fibre is essential to the efficient working of the digestive system.

🌑 **Call the doctor**

*If pain becomes more severe, is associated with a fever or has lasted more than a day or two; if you are in severe pain and unable to hold down fluids for more than 12 hours; if a child has severe abdominal pain.*

# Flatulence

*Excessive wind, either through the mouth or through the anus, as a by-product of the digestive process; often associated with a bloated feeling in the abdomen.*

PEAS

omedians joke about it, yet nothing could be more natural than flatulence – the normal by-product of digestion and fermentation that takes place in the gut. Many people feel obsessive anxiety about flatulence, but unless it becomes excessive there is no need for concern. Any sudden change in the everyday build-up and release of these gases could, however, herald an underlying problem. Possible causes are hiatus hernia, Irritable Bowel Syndrome *(see p.94)*, diverticulitis or severe constipation *(see p.96)*. But in the absence of other disease, home remedies will usually overcome this problem.

**BELOW** Small changes in diet can bring about relief from excessive flatulence.

## CONVENTIONAL MEDICINE

A change in diet can be helpful, cutting down on pulses, such as beans and lentils. Other foods that could be reduced include brussels sprouts, peas, cabbage and eggs. If the problem persists, try taking an antacid that contains dimethicone.

SPROUTS

DOSAGE: ADULTS AND CHILDREN Many suitable preparations are available to help with flatulence, either as tablets or in liquid form; consult pack for details, or follow medical advice.

## HERBAL REMEDIES

There is a wide choice of herbal carminatives to dispel gas in the digestive tract and improve function. The range includes aniseed, cardamom, cayenne (chilli), cinnamon, clove, coriander, garlic, ginger, nutmeg, sage and thyme.

USE AND DOSAGE Adding these herbs to cooking is an easy way to avoid digestive problems. Alternatively, drink them in infusions or try teas of camomile, holy thistle, lemon balm or peppermint after meals.

## HOMEOPATHIC REMEDIES

꩜ Raphanus 6c

For flatulence after abdominal operations when wind feels trapped. Distended abdomen, colicky pains.

꩜ Carbo vegetabilis 6c

For heaviness after meals, sleepiness and belching. Flatus smells offensive. Craves sweet and salt foods.

DOSAGE 1 tablet hourly for six doses, then twice daily. Maximum 1 week.

## AROMATHERAPY

꩜ Roman camomile (Chamaemelum nobile)

꩜ Fennel (Foeniculum vulgare)

꩜ Ginger (Zingiber officinale)

꩜ Marjoram (Origanum majorana)

꩜ Peppermint (Mentha x piperita)

These oils aid gas dispersal and soothe the pain associated with flatulence.

APPLICATION Use in either an oil-based or lotion-based massage and rub onto the abdomen.

## NUTRITION

In order to prevent flatulence you must allow time for the digestive process to work – so savour your food and chew it well. Avoid all carbonated drinks and reduce your consumption of sugar in all forms; also avoid foods like beans, brussels sprouts, cauliflower and other 'windy' foods if you are suffering from flatulence. But as your eating habits improve and you add to your diet more live yogurt and other fermented milk products, with all their beneficial bacteria, you will find that you can return to eating virtually anything. It helps, too, if you add caraway seeds when cooking cabbage, and summer savory to all bean dishes. Dill – both seeds and fronds (the leaves) – fennel seeds, licorice, parsley and mint can all be added to cooking and taken as tea, both to prevent and relieve excessive wind.

Constipation (see p.96) is an extremely common cause of wind and will be exacerbated if you start adding bran to your daily food intake. Instead, eat foods that contain soluble fibre, such as oats.

### Prevention

*Food combining, also known as the Hay diet (see p.200), which involves separating protein foods (like meat, fish, cheese and eggs) from starchy foods (like bread, potatoes, rice, pasta, cereals, biscuits and cakes), may be a long-term solution for some people suffering from flatulence.*

GOAT'S CHEESE

BREAD

**ABOVE** Food combining may help: its principles state that bread and cheese should not be eaten together, but neutral foods like peas and lentils can be eaten with anything.

# Gall-bladder problems

*Gallstones may not produce any symptoms, but can cause recurrent, painful attacks in the upper right abdomen; jaundice, with the whites of the eyes and skin appearing yellow; pain associated with fever; nausea is common.*

The risk factors for the developments of gallstones are obesity, increasing age and female gender (and women are twice as likely as men to get them). At their worst, gallstones can block the flow of bile from the gall bladder to the stomach and, without bile, the digestion of fats becomes almost impossible. Then the sometimes horrendous symptoms of projectile vomiting and violent pain may ensue. However, home remedies can prevent problems recurring.

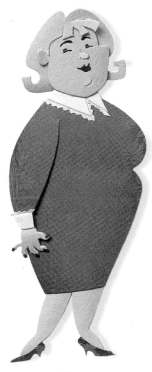

**ABOVE** Women are much more likely than men to be susceptible to gallstones.

### CONVENTIONAL MEDICINE

If the pain from a gallstone continues, despite taking pain relievers, contact a doctor. Seek immediate medical help if it is associated with fever or jaundice. **DOSAGE: ADULTS** 1–2 tablets of pain relievers at onset of pain, repeated every 4 hours; consult pack.

### HERBAL REMEDIES

Professional help is essential for severe or persistent problems, but general discomfort can be soothed by anti-inflammatory and bitter herbs.
**USE AND DOSAGE** Try the 'olive oil and lemon' remedy for gallstones: after breakfast eat nothing more until early evening, then drink 30–60ml/1–2fl oz of olive oil, followed by the juice of 1–2 lemons diluted with as little warm water as possible. Alternate this combination every 20–30 minutes through the evening until you have consumed 500ml/18fl oz of olive oil and the juice of about 9–10 lemons. The gallstones should then be passed, as small stones and gritty sand with stools, over the next 3 days.

Try decoctions of milk-thistle seeds, fringe-tree bark or wild-yam root (1tsp per cup), or an infusion of fumitory and agrimony (1tsp each per cup).

Bitters before meals (2–5 drops of gentian, wormwood or centaury tincture) encourage bile flow.

## HOMEOPATHIC REMEDIES

Consult a doctor for gall-bladder problems.

**Chelidonium 6c**

For pain under right ribs extending to right shoulder blade. Colic, jaundice, gallstones, 'bilious vomiting'. Stools pasty/yellow.

**Berberis 6c**

For pain under right ribs radiating to stomach and all over body. Worse for pressure. Watery stools that are clay-coloured.

**Hydrastis 6c**

For gallstones, tenderness over liver. No appetite or thirst. Jaundice. Stools white.

DOSAGE 1 tablet every 2–3 hours for six doses, then three times daily for 2–3 days.

## AROMATHERAPY

**Lavender** (*Lavandula angustifolia*)

**Roman camomile** (*Chamaemelum nobile*)

These oils help to reduce the pain.

APPLICATION Use in a massage oil or lotion, then apply over the area of the gall bladder.

## NUTRITION

A problematic gall bladder necessitates quite a strict food regime. Eat plenty of vegetables, fruit and wholegrain cereals (particularly oats); plenty of fish, (but avoid smoked fish); and beans. Have at least one large garlic clove (or a high-strength garlic pill) daily. Try to eat fresh globe artichokes at least two or three times a week – its chemicals have a specific stimulating effect on the gall bladder and liver.

Avoid alcohol and caffeine, but drink a minimum of 1.7l/3pt of water, in addition to other drinks, daily. Avoid all animal fats (no beef, pork or lamb, duck or goose). Roasted (unbasted), grilled or boiled chicken without skin is all right. Eat no butter, cream, cheese (except cottage cheese), eggs or fried food. You can use skimmed milk, very low-fat yogurt and a little olive, sunflower or safflower oil. Do not eat sausages, salami, pâté, ham, bacon, meat pies, pasties or any processed meat.

### Call the doctor

*If pain persists, especially if there is jaundice, a raised temperature or protracted vomiting.*

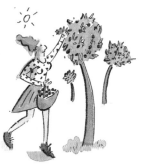

### Caution

*Always read pain-reliever packages carefully, and do not exceed the stated dose.*

BELOW Salmon can be a part of the strict diet necessary with gall-bladder problems.

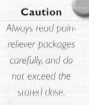

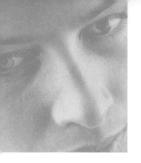

# Infestation:
## worms and parasites

*Parasitic skin infections may be characterized by an itchy rash; worms in the digestive tract may be passed in the stool and cause itching around the anus.*

Parasites like headlice and scabies and the wide variety of intestinal worms, such as threadworm, are no respecters of person or position. Intestinal parasites require medical attention, while skin infestations can take several treatments to clear, particularly in the case of headlice, which have become resistant to some currently available medicated shampoos and treatment lotions.

### Call the doctor

*If you suspect that you are suffering from an intestinal parasite.*

### Prevention

*Most worms survive only in raw or undercooked food, so try to eat properly cooked food when abroad. The only way to protect yourself against headlice is never to let your hair come into direct contact with anyone else's.*

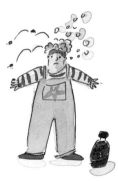

### CONVENTIONAL MEDICINE

Threadworms are easily treated with a single dose of mebendazole, but make sure you treat the whole family. Parasitic skin infestations can be treated with insecticides, available as lotions and shampoos (treat the whole affected area). Do not use insecticides too frequently on children; instead, for headlice, try regularly combing the hair with a fine nit-comb after washing. Apply conditioner and leave for 5 minutes before combing, then wash off.

DOSAGE: ADULTS AND CHILDREN For scabies, apply a water-based solution all over the body.

For headlice, apply a water-based lotion to the whole scalp. Repeat after 7 days.

For threadworms, take one dose of mebendazole, repeated 2 weeks later.

### HERBAL REMEDIES

Cabbage is a traditional remedy for threadworms and can be used like carrots *(see under Nutrition)*. Take garlic as a preventative when travelling.

USE AND DOSAGE Wormwood is effective, but is very bitter: 5ml/1tsp (1ml/¼tsp for children) of the tincture, well diluted in water or carrot juice and taken on an empty stomach, may be sufficient to clear the problem. Repeat after 14 days (to match the threadworm's life cycle).

## ❖ HOMEOPATHIC REMEDIES

The following remedies should help to clear worms. If the symptoms persist, consult a doctor.

#### Cina 6c

Common name: wormseed. For patient who is restless and irritable. Itchy rectum. May have diarrhoea and cramping abdominal pain, better for pressure.

#### Sabadilla 6c

For chilly and not thirsty person. Itching in the rectum may alternate with itchy nose.

DOSAGE 1 tablet twice daily. Maximum 1 week.

#### Staphysagria

For headlice, dilute mother tincture (available at homeopathic pharmacies) in a ratio of 1:10 with baby shampoo. Shampoo the hair, then leave on for 10 minutes, rinse and comb hair through. Repeat next night if there are further signs of lice. Repeat again 1 week later.

### Caution

*Asthmatics should avoid using alcoholic solutions for headlice; the same thing applies to infants.*

## AROMATHERAPY

- Rosemary (Rosmarinus officinalis)
- Lavender (Lavandula angustifolia)
- Roman camomile (Chamaemelum nobile)
- Niaouli (Melaleuca viridiflora)
- Eucalyptus (Eucalyptus radiata)
- Tea tree (Melaleuca alternifolia)

These oils are soothing and help to fight infection.

APPLICATION For threadworm, massage the oils into the abdomen. This should be accompanied by treatment from your doctor or pharmacist. For headlice, add 1–2 drops of the oils to the final rinse water; or mix 2–3 drops with some warm vegetable oil (about 5ml/1tsp), then massage into the hair, wrap the hair in clingfilm and a warm towel, and leave overnight. In the morning comb through, then wash out the hair; repeat if necessary.

## NUTRITION

Eat a big portion of carrots or drink a large glass of carrot juice each day, to treat worms. Additionally, drink the juice of a whole lemon vigorously mixed with 15ml/1tbsp of olive oil.

# Peptic ulcers

*Characterized by pain in the upper abdomen, often in a specific place, which may be pointed out with one finger; pain is often worse at night; it may also be worse when hungry and associated with nausea, flatulence and heartburn.*

Peptic ulcers are caused by erosion of the lining of the stomach by excessive amounts of gastric acid. While stress frequently plays a part, we now know that the balance between the acid digestive juices and the protective mucus produced by the stomach lining is also upset. The latest research has shown that bacteria called *Helicobacter pylori* may cause some ulcers. These bacteria are very widespread and are common in cats, which may pass them on to their human owners.

## 🌐 Call the doctor

*If you have specific pain in the upper abdomen and have lost weight unintentionally; if it is the first time you have had these symptoms and you are over 40 years old; if the pain persists, despite symptomatic measures.*

### ✚ CONVENTIONAL MEDICINE

Avoid spicy foods, hot drinks, alcohol and smoking. Do not take NSAIDs, which are often used for pain relief. Eat frequent, regular small meals of bland food. Antacids may help if symptoms persist for more than a week. Be aware they usually contain magnesium or aluminium salts: the former (e.g. Milk of Magnesia) tend to cause diarrhoea; the latter (e.g. Aluminium hydroxide) constipation. Your doctor may refer you for further tests or recommend a trial of an $H2$ antagonist. If you have *Helicobacter pylori* infection, you may need antibiotics.

Dosage: Adults and children over 16 Many types of antacid are available as tablets or in liquid form; consult pack for details.

### ▨ HERBAL REMEDIES

Try herbal antibacterials, such as blue flag, echinacea, red clover, thyme and wild indigo, in capsules or teas to combat the underlying cause. Symptomatic relief comes from soothing demulcents, like slippery elm or marsh-mallow, meadowsweet or Irish moss, taken as teas, liquid extracts or tinctures.

Use and Dosage Make 2tsp of slippery-elm powder into a gruel with a cup of hot milk.

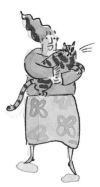

Make a strong decoction of licorice root, or dissolve licorice-juice sticks in water and take in 10ml/2tsp doses or add to teas.

### ✿ HOMEOPATHIC REMEDIES

A consultation with a homeopath is recommended, after seeing your doctor.

#### ✑ Arsenicum album 6c

For raw, burning feeling in stomach. Worse for food and drink. Better for milk. Food feels as if it sticks in gullet, with nothing going through. Person is frightened and restless.

#### ✑ Phosphorus 6c

For burning pain. Worse for eating, better for cold food. Thirst for ice-cold water, but vomits soon afterwards. May vomit 'coffee grounds'.

DOSAGE  1 tablet twice daily. Maximum 2 weeks.

**ABOVE** A kiwi fruit contains twice as much vitamin C as an orange.

> **Caution**
> Non-steroidal anti-inflammatory drugs (NSAIDs) can make the symptoms worse.

### 🍎 NUTRITION

Eat plenty of wholegrains, pumpkin seeds, oysters and most shellfish for their zinc; broccoli, red and green peppers, kiwis, apricots and the sweeter citrus fruit for their vitamin C and beta-carotene; oily fish for its omega-3 fatty acids, which protect the whole gastric lining. A diet that is rich in fibre is also protective, but avoid spoonfuls of uncooked bran. Oats, brown rice and most root vegetables contain soluble fibre, which is more soothing.

Scientists in New Zealand have shown that manuka honey (from the tea tree) can kill the bug responsible for ulcers. A dessertspoon with each meal and another at bedtime will normally produce results within a few weeks. In European natural medicine, raw cabbage and potato juice are known to be effective – take a small wine glass before each meal, on a daily alternating basis.

### 💧 AROMATHERAPY

The aim of aromatherapy here is to reduce stress levels, rather than treat the ulcer. So look up the oils for stress (see p.36). Make sure that you get a good diagnosis and do truly have a peptic ulcer.

# Irritable bowel syndrome: IBS

*Recurrent episodes of abdominal pain with constipation or diarrhoea; the pain is often relieved by passing wind or a bowel movement.*

**I**rritable bowel syndrome has in recent years graduated from a relatively obscure condition, known as spastic colon, to epidemic proportions throughout Britain and the US. Though it can be the sequel to a severe bout of food poisoning or gastroenteritis, it is far more likely to be the result of an over-consumption of bran fibre and under-consumption of the soluble fibre that is found in fruit and vegetables. It is not caused by the yeast infection *Candida*; nor is it, as many doctors believe, a symptom of depression or other psychological illness. Stress, however, can play a major part.

**BELOW** Anti-spasmodic drugs can alleviate the symptoms of IBS, but dietary changes will also be needed.

### CONVENTIONAL MEDICINE

Keeping a food diary can help to establish links between symptoms and particular foods. Relaxation techniques may be beneficial. If the symptoms persist, your doctor may recommend medication to relax the muscle in the digestive tract.

### HERBAL REMEDIES

Herbs can help ease the discomfort.

USE AND DOSAGE Make an infusion from equal amounts of agrimony, hops, meadowsweet and peppermint and drink a cup before meals.

Simmer 2tsp of fenugreek seeds with a pinch of cinnamon in water for 10–15 minutes, then drink.

Herbs like wild yam and cramp bark can ease painful gut spasms and cramps: use in decoctions or as tinctures (10 drops taken on the tongue at 30-minute intervals).

### HOMEOPATHIC REMEDIES

If the following do not help, consult a homeopath.

**Lycopodium 6c**

For bloating, better for passing wind. Rumbling in stomach. Eating little gives a sense of fullness.

Craves sweets, warm food and drink. Hard stool changes to liquid. Constipation away from home.

 Nux vomica 6c

For cramping abdominal pains. Worse for eating. Better after the bowels open and for warm drinks. Constipation: small amounts of stool. Constant feeling of need to go to toilet. Diarrhoea alternates with constipation.

DOSAGE 1 tablet twice daily. Maximum 1 week.

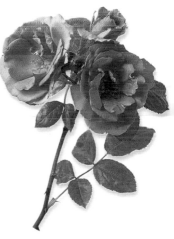

ABOVE A craving for sweets is a symptom of some types of IBS.

## AROMATHERAPY

 Neroli *(Citrus aurantium)*

 Roman camomile *(Chamaemelum nobile)*

 Rose *(Rosa damascena/Rosa centifolia)*

These oils are calming and soothing.

APPLICATION Use in abdominal massage, with either an aqueous cream or oil. These oils can also be used in a warm compress or in the bath.

## NUTRITION

If alternating bouts of constipation, diarrhoea, flatulence and stomach distension have been with you for years, do not despair. Changing your eating habits can restore your life to normal. Keep detailed records of what you eat and its effects, so that you know which foods are okay and which to avoid.

Eat plenty of food that contains soluble fibre – fruit, vegetables, beans and especially oats. Cereals contain a mixture of soluble and insoluble fibre; wheat bran is not only an irritant, but can interfere with the way the body absorbs vital nutrients like iron and calcium. You must drink at least 1.5l/2½pt of water every day and ensure that you eat proper meals at regular intervals. Make generous use of all the herbs that help the digestive process – rosemary, sage, thyme, mint, dill, caraway, garlic and ginger.

For some people IBS is an adverse reaction to specific foods. These (in descending order of likelihood) are: meat and meat products, dairy produce and wheat products. Try excluding them in groups – one at a time, for at least 2 weeks to provide clues about which foods to avoid.

### Prevention

*Simple herbal remedies like hypericum have no side-effects and are not habit-forming and will help with depression while you experiment with your diet.*

ABOVE Rose oil used in an abdominal massage can help to soothe pain and discomfort.

# Constipation

*Typified by a straining to defecate; hard faeces that are sometimes painful to pass; stomach pain, bloating and wind; and a general feeling of malaise.*

PRUNES

onstipation is one of the most common digestive problems, and the one that is most suited to home treatment. People vary as to how often they open their bowels: some maybe no more than every 2 or 3 days; others two or three times a day, or more often. Children, the elderly and pregnant women are more prone to constipation, but it can occur in either sex at any age. A lack of the right sort of soluble fibre, insufficient fluid and bad toilet habits are the prime causes.

## CONVENTIONAL MEDICINE

If the bowel has stretched and is full of faeces, it needs retraining to respond to the urge to go to the toilet regularly, without straining. Changing your diet and increasing your fluid intake may take a day or two to have any effect. In the meantime, a laxative and suppositories can help. If you suspect that prescribed medicines are causing your constipation, consult your doctor before reducing the dose. If constipation persists seek medical help.

DOSAGE: ADULTS Natural or vegetable laxatives are safe and non-addictive, so ask your pharmacist for advice; consult pack for dosage information. One or two glycerol suppositories once a day, moistened before use, will stimulate bowel movement.

DOSAGE: CHILDREN See a doctor before giving laxatives.

## HERBAL REMEDIES

Drastic herbal purgatives – like senna and cascara sagrada – should only be used in moderation.

USE AND DOSAGE Each morning take a decoction of equal amounts of dandelion, yellow dock and licorice roots (2tsp to 1½ cups of water, simmered for 10 minutes) with a pinch of anise or fennel seeds to ease griping.

Lubricate the bowel with ispaghula seeds – add 1tsp to a cup of boiling water, allow to cool, then drink; orange juice instead of water improves the flavour.

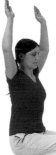

**LEFT** Sit tall with your legs straight out in front of you, then raise your arms above your head.

## ✿ HOMEOPATHIC REMEDIES

Sudden changes in bowel habit need medical attention.

### ᦈ Alumina 6c

For soft, sticky or hard, dry stools that are difficult to pass, even when soft. Constipation in the elderly, from inactivity. No urge to open bowels.

### ᦈ Bryonia 6c

For hard, dry, large crumbly stools. May have diarrhoea after taking cold drinks. Thirsty for large quantities of fluids.

**DOSAGE** 1 tablet three times daily Maximum 1 week.

**BELOW** Exhale and bend forwards towards your feet, then lower your head and hold for several breaths.

## NUTRITION

Drink at least 2l/3½pt of water each day and eat unpeeled apples, pears, root vegetables, oats, beans and all green vegetables; at least one carton of live natural yogurt daily; and plenty of real wholemeal bread. Brown rice, wholewheat pasta, porridge and muesli are great providers of soluble fibre. Do not use uncooked bran or high-bran cereals.

For a gentle laxative pour 1.2l/2pt of boiling water over 1kg/2lb of stoned prunes and a few pieces of bruised licorice stick. Leave to stand overnight. Remove the licorice, then purée the prunes in a liquidizer. Keep in the refrigerator and take two dessertspoons with breakfast and two with a warm drink at bedtime.

**LEFT** Sit with your left arm around your right knee, with your right hand on the floor behind you.

## AROMATHERAPY

ᦈ Black pepper *(Piper nigrum)*
ᦈ Ginger *(Zingiber officinale)*
ᦈ Marjoram *(Origanum majorana)*

These oils stimulate the digestive system.

**APPLICATION** Mix the essential oil with either a lotion or a carrier oil and massage over the abdomen in a clockwise direction.

**LEFT** Breathe out and turn to look behind you. Hold for several breaths, then repeat on the other side.

# Diarrhoea

*Passing of faeces more frequently, which are often soft or watery, or may be more bulky than usual; there may also be symptoms reflecting the underlying cause of the diarrhoea, including fever, vomiting and crampy abdominal pain.*

**D**iarrhoea is a symptom, not an illness. The passing of frequent, loose or even liquid stool (sometimes uncontrollable) is the result of irritation or inflammation of the gut. It is often accompanied by severe vomiting and may be caused by overindulgence, too much alcohol or by bacterial infection from food poisoning. Most minor bouts can be dealt with adequately at home, but prolonged diarrhoea may be the result of a more serious underlying illness and can cause severe dehydration, particularly in small children and the elderly.

## 🌐 Call the doctor

*If there is any sudden change in bowel habits that lasts more than 2–3 days (sooner in children and the elderly).*

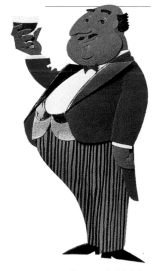

**ABOVE** Too much rich living can bring on an attack of diarrhoea.

### ✚ CONVENTIONAL MEDICINE

Water, salts and minerals lost through diarrhoea need to be replaced. This is particularly important in children and frail adults. Drinking extra water will help, but special oral rehydration fluid preparations are available. They can be flavoured or made into ice cubes to make them more palatable. Prolonged diarrhoea may require medical treatment, especially if there is blood, severe abdominal pain or high fever. DOSAGE: ADULTS AND CHILDREN Dissolve the contents of an oral rehydration sachet in water and drink after each episode of diarrhoea. Consult pack.

### HERBAL REMEDIES

To soothe an inflamed digestive tract, drink unsweetened black tea: the high tannin content soothes and repairs sore tissues. Other herbs to use in teas include agrimony, bistort, lady's mantle, meadowsweet, raspberry leaves and tormentil. USE AND DOSAGE Use 2tsp of herb per cup of boiling water.

Pack a small bottle of tincture of any of these herbs to combat holiday diarrhoea (take 5ml/1tsp in water up to six times a day), or eat pawpaw – a traditional tropical remedy.

### HOMEOPATHIC REMEDIES

Diarrhoea requires the same general measures as for gastroenteritis *(see p.102).* Persistent diarrhoea needs medical investigation.

**Podophyllum 6c**
Gushing, watery diarrhoea; flatus sometimes causes stool to pass. Stool offensive, may be pasty or yellow. Colic pains before stool better for lying on abdomen.

**China 6c**
For painless diarrhoea of undigested food, flatulence and colic. Worse after eating fruit. Patient feels weak.
**Dosage** 1 tablet hourly until improved, then every 4 hours. Maximum 5 days.

### NUTRITION

Unless absolutely essential, do not take anti-diarrhoea drugs for the first 24 hours and do not eat, either. You must replace fluids and electrolytes, so make up 1l/1¾pt of freshly boiled water with a mixture of 8tsp of sugar and 1tsp of salt, and drink the whole amount at least twice a day. After 24 hours use the BRAT diet: ripe Bananas, boiled Rice, Apples and dry wholemeal Toast. Eat little and often for the next 48 hours, then add boiled or jacket potatoes, cooked carrots with other mixed vegetables, and an egg. Gradually get back to normal eating, saving all dairy products until last.

To relieve diarrhoea, crush four cloves of garlic and stir into a 450g/1lb jar of honey. Dissolve a dessertspoon in a tumbler of hot water and sip slowly, repeating three times daily.

### AROMATHERAPY

**Roman camomile** *(Chamaemelum nobile)*
**Neroli** *(Citrus aurantium)*
**Lavender** *(Lavandula angustifolia)*
**Peppermint** *(Mentha piperita)*
These oils are antispasmodic and help griping stomach pains. They are also soothing to the digestive tract and nervous system. Camomile is an anti-allergen, useful if the diarrhoea is an allergic reaction.
**Application** Apply gentle abdominal massage.

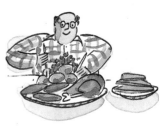

> **Caution**
> *Avoid medicines that claim to stop diarrhoea, as they tend to prolong the illness. Reserve them for occasions when it may be hard to use a toilet frequently, such as while you are travelling.*

**BELOW** Components of the BRAT diet: Banana, Rice, Apple, Toast.

# Weight problems

*Difficulty in maintaining your weight at that expected for your height and build; you may weigh either more or less than your ideal weight, or it may fluctuate from one to the other; neither extreme of the weight spectrum is healthy.*

The Western world is obsessed with being overweight, but the real truth is that diets often do not work in the long term. At the other end of the scale there are many thousands of people desperate to gain weight. Being severely overweight increases the risk of heart disease, diabetes, respiratory problems, arthritis and some forms of cancer; being painfully thin increases the risk of osteoporosis, menstrual problems and reduced life expectancy. The overweight will only achieve long-term success by changing the way they eat and increasing their exercise; the skinnies by eating high-energy foods more frequently.

## Call the doctor

*If you are seriously concerned about your weight.*

## CONVENTIONAL MEDICINE

To lose weight, eat smaller portions of everything, avoiding fatty and sugary food and excessive amounts of alcohol. In order to gain weight, do the reverse, but do not increase the amount of alcohol that you consume or food containing high amounts of sugar. Treating a serious weight problem may require qualified dietary advice. Psychological help is beneficial in some severe cases.

## HERBAL REMEDIES

Herbal remedies are no real substitute for calorie control, healthy eating and regular exercise, and any proprietary 'slimming' tea should be regarded with suspicion: many are mixtures of strong laxatives and diuretics, which will have only a short-term effect on weight problems. Kelp can be useful, if the weight problem is associated with a sluggish metabolism or an underactive thyroid, although professional help is generally advisable in such cases. Malabar tamarind is sometimes recommended as a useful treatment for short-term use, as it affects carbohydrate metabolism and can therefore help to prevent overeating.

### ❖ HOMEOPATHIC REMEDIES

Best treated with a remedy specific to the individual, so consult a qualified homeopath if possible.

#### ☙ Sulphur 30c

For plump, hearty person with red cheeks. Lazy, untidy, does not feel the cold and is worse for heat. Very sweaty, with hot feet, put out of bed at night.

#### ☙ Calcarea carbonica 30c

For flabby person, who puts on weight easily. Soft face, pale complexion. Sweaty head at night. Chilly, cold. Cold feet at night in bed and wants to wear socks, removed when feet get too hot.

**DOSAGE** 1 tablet twice daily. Maximum 1 week.

### ◐ AROMATHERAPY

People with weight problems often have a very poor self-image, for which useful oils would be jasmine, frankincense and sandalwood. Any citrus or floral oil will help the accompanying depression. Use the oils in a way that supports you – in the bath, in massage, as a perfume; as a lotion for your face, body or hands; or just a drop on your clothes.

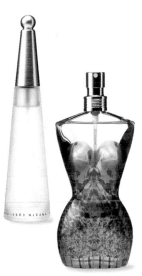

**ABOVE** Choose a perfume that lifts your mood and improves your self-image.

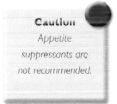

**Caution**
Appetite suppressants are not recommended.

### ◑ NUTRITION

There is only one successful route to weight loss and that is to change your eating habits. Balanced consumption of real food eaten at proper intervals, combined with some exercise, is the only remedy that works. So eat plenty of good carbohydrates, such as brown rice, potatoes, wholemeal bread, beans and pasta, fresh vegetables, fruit and salads, fish and skinless poultry. Remember: if you have one bad meal, or even a bad week, don't quit; just get yourself back on track as soon as possible.

Those of you desperately trying to gain weight have to increase your calorie consumption without relying on high-fat meat and dairy products. Good carbohydrates (see above) are excellent sources of calories, but bulky. Eat modest amounts of food, but at least every 2–3 hours. Get extra calories from fresh unsalted nuts, seeds, unsalted peanut butter, tahini, avocados, olive oil and dried fruit.

BROWN RICE

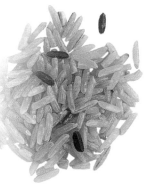

# Gastroenteritis,
## including food poisoning

*Characterized by nausea and vomiting, which may be severe; diarrhoea, often quite acute; crampy abdominal pain; and mild fever.*

**A**cute and violent diarrhoea and vomiting may be caused by an infection, but acute gastroenteritis is most commonly caused by food poisoning transmitted by food that has spoiled, been improperly cooked or handled. For an otherwise fit and healthy adult, home remedies can help bring about rapid recovery.

### CONVENTIONAL MEDICINE

Take a sip of fluid every 5 minutes. If the vomiting continues and symptoms persist for more than 12 hours, seek urgent medical attention. For less severe symptoms, drinking extra water will help, but special oral rehydration fluid preparations are available, tasting like strong mineral water. Prolonged diarrhoea may require further treatment, so seek medical advice.

**DOSAGE: ADULTS AND CHILDREN** Dissolve the contents of an oral rehydration sachet in water and drink after each episode of diarrhoea; consult pack for details.

### 🌙 Call the doctor

*If diarrhoea or vomiting is prolonged, to rule out any underlying illness; if you have been unable to hold down fluids for longer than 12 hours; if there is associated blood or high fever.*

### HERBAL REMEDIES

Herbs can ease the symptoms, while nature gets rid of the irritant.

**USE AND DOSAGE** Combine bistort and fenugreek decoction with an agrimony and gotu kola infusion (1 cup of the mixture, three to five times daily) to soothe the lower bowel.

Take slippery elm or marsh-mallow capsules to protect the gut lining. Bilberry or cranberry juice combats fluid loss while easing bowel discomfort.

*Aloe vera* juice is an ideal remedy, if available.

Take 10 drops of echinacea tincture in a little water every few hours in order to combat any infecting organisms.

## ✿ HOMEOPATHIC REMEDIES

Starve for 24 hours, maintaining hydration with sips of water every 15 minutes. The following remedy may be used for travellers' diarrhoea.

### ❧ Arsenicum album 6c

For gastroenteritis from food poisoning. Diarrhoea and vomiting at the same time. Chilly, better for warmth. Patient restless, anxious, weak. Heat improves burning abdominal pain. Thirsty for sips of liquid.

**DOSAGE** 1 tablet hourly until improved, then every 4 hours. Maximum 5 days.

## AROMATHERAPY

- ❧ Roman camomile *(Chamaemelum nobile)*
- ❧ Lavender *(Lavandula angustifolia)*
- ❧ Melissa *(Melissa officinalis)*
- ❧ Tea tree *(Melaleuca alternifolia)*

Tea tree is antiviral and antibacterial. Camomile and lavender are soothing and painkilling. Melissa is anti-depressant and relieves spasms in the digestive tract.

**APPLICATION** Tea tree is useful in the home, especially to protect other members of the family – so burn it, and use it to wash all surfaces down, wash out the bath and any soiled linen. Use the other oils in the bath, in body lotion or for massage.

## NUTRITION

The first step is always to replace lost fluids and electrolytes (see Diarrhoea on p.98). You will not feel like eating until the worst symptoms have abated. When you do, avoid all dairy products for at least 48 hours and stick to the BRAT diet – ripe Bananas, boiled Rice, Apples and dry wholemeal Toast (see p.99). Do not have any ice-cold drinks and avoid all citrus juices.

Yogurt plays a vital role in recovering from gastro-enteritis. Its natural bacteria destroy unwelcome bacteria in the gut and have an immune-boosting effect. This is also true of fermented milk products. Unfortunately, none of these benefits is provided by most commercial yogurts, so you must choose live yogurt, a rich source of beneficial probiotic bacteria.

CAMOMILE

### Caution

Severe gastroenteritis, especially in children or the elderly, may be extremely grave. Avoid medicines that claim to stop diarrhoea, as they tend to prolong the illness; reserve them for occasions when it may be hard to use a toilet frequently

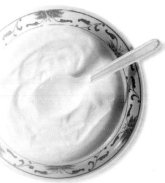

**BELOW** A portion of live yogurt will soothe the gut and boost the immune system.

# Gastritis

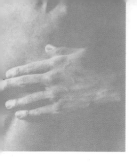

*Pain or discomfort in the upper abdomen, related to food; may be associated with nausea or burping.*

Severe and sudden gastritis – or inflammation of the stomach lining – is nearly always self-inflicted. Too much alcohol, too many cigarettes, very hot curries and even some medicines can all act as the trigger.

## 🌐 Call the doctor

*If the symptoms persist or if they are not relieved by antacids.*

**BELOW** A herbal infusion can help to relieve the pain of gastritis.

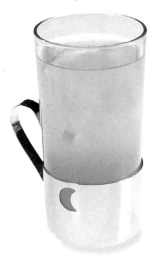

### ✚ CONVENTIONAL MEDICINE

Avoid NSAIDs, which are often taken for pain relief. Frequent small meals of bland food may relieve the symptoms. Antacids can also be helpful *(see p.78).*

### ▱ HERBAL REMEDIES

USE AND DOSAGE Take slippery elm or marsh-mallow as tablets or as powders, made into a paste with warm water.

Fenugreek seeds (2tsp per cup) in a decoction with a pinch of powdered cinnamon can bring relief; or use lemon balm, meadowsweet and fennel in an infusion (½–1tsp of each per cup).

Use licorice root in a decoction or dissolve 2.5cm/1in of a licorice stick in a cup of hot water.

### ✽ HOMEOPATHIC REMEDIES

Severe or persistent pains, or vomiting blood or dark fluid, require medical attention. A consultation with a qualified homeopath is recommended.

🔹 **Nux vomica 6c**

For gastritis from alcohol. Cannot stand pressure around waist. Cramping pains, worse for eating, anger. Workaholic and irritable.

🔹 **Capsicum 6c**

For burning or icy-cold feeling in stomach. Wants coffee but makes them nauseous. Lots of flatulence.

DOSAGE 1 tablet taken every 2 hours for six doses, then three times daily. Maximum 3 days.

# The Reproductive System

The average woman will have about 400 menstrual periods during her life, which are regulated by hormones in the bloodstream. Although the hormonal level varies during the course of the cycle, if there is any upset in the balance of the hormones, then menstrual disorders, **PMS** and menopausal problems may occur. But help is at hand in the form of nutritional supplements and healthy eating, as well as hormone-balancing herbs, de-stressing oils and homeopathic remedies.

# Menstrual problems

*Too frequent, irregular or absent periods (amenorrhoea); painful periods (dysmenorrhoea); periods that last an exceptionally long time; heavy periods (menorrhagia), possibly with clots.*

**The menstrual cycle is controlled by your body's production of hormones and anything that interferes with this mechanism – significant loss or gain of weight, stress, anxiety or depression – will affect your periods. The underlying causes of menstrual disorder may be simple and medically unimportant, or complex and carry serious medical implications, but home remedies can play an important part in resolving many of them. (See also Osteoporosis on p.70, Menopause on p.110, Fibroids on p.114 and PMS on p.108).**

### CONVENTIONAL MEDICINE

Most changes in the menstrual cycle are transient, but if there has been a sustained change for more than 6 months, your doctor may wish to investigate. Painful periods may need investigation, but can often be treated with prescribed pain relievers containing mefenamic acid, which also helps to reduce the amount of blood. The commonest reason for a missed period is pregnancy. Excessive weight loss and exercise can both stop periods occurring.

### HOMEOPATHIC REMEDIES

It is useful to consult a qualified homeopath.

**Magnesium phosphate 30c**

For colicky abdominal pains, eased by hot-water bottle and pressing firmly on abdomen. Better when period is flowing.

**Cimicifuga racemosa 30c**

For labour-like pains from hip to hip. Worse for movement. Pains worse, the heavier the period. Better for bending double. Person is chilly and thirsty.

**Sepia 30c**

For cramping, heavy pains in uterus. Better for sitting with crossed legs. Tired.

**DOSAGE** I tablet 2–4 hourly. Maximum 12 doses.

**Call the doctor**
*If you are having long-term or very uncomfortable menstrual problems.*

### HERBAL REMEDIES

Warming herbal teas help soothe period pain.

**USE AND DOSAGE** Mix equal amounts of St John's wort, raspberry leaves and skullcap (2tsp per cup).

Black haw helps relax cramping pains: take 20ml/4tsp of the tincture as a single dose in warm water; repeat after 4 hours if necessary.

For heavy periods use a tea of lady's mantle, shepherd's purse and marigold (2tsp of each per cup).

Agnus-castus is a hormone regulator: use 20 drops of tincture in water each morning.

**ABOVE** Marigold can be combined with shepherd's purse and lady's mantle to relieve heavy periods.

### NUTRITION

What you eat and drink plays a vital part in the solution of all menstrual problems. Eat plenty of wholegrain cereals, yeast extracts, wheatgerm, dried fruit, nuts, bananas and oats for their vitamin B; oily fish for its essential fatty acids; cold-pressed oils, wheatgerm, avocados and all edible seeds for their vitamin E. Get lots of zinc (from shellfish, sardines, pumpkin seeds and peas) and selenium (from wholemeal bread, brazil nuts, almonds and soya products). Add some borage flowers to salad to help relieve the discomfort of menstrual problems.

If you are constantly dieting, your weight is going down and your periods are irregular, you may be heading for anorexia and an artificially induced menopause. Heavy periods increase the risk of iron deficiency and anaemia, so eat more of the foods rich in iron, including liver (but not if you are pregnant), dark green leafy vegetables, raisins, dates, watercress and eggs.

RAISINS

### AROMATHERAPY

- Rose *(Rosa damascena/Rosa centifolia)*
- Geranium *(Pelargonium graveolens)*
- Clary sage *(Salvia sclarea)*

These oils relate to the feminine aspect and help women feel they are in control of their own bodies.

**APPLICATION** Use in the bath, in massage oil or lotion, or as a compress.

### Prevention

*Try to avoid constipation (see p.96), which can cause pressure on the abdomen and aggravate menstrual problems. So eat plenty of soluble and insoluble fibre (but avoid bran) and drink at least 2.75l/5pt of liquid each day.*

*An excess of alcohol or caffeine may interfere with blood flow to the uterus and lead to menstrual difficulties, while salt can be a major hazard, since it leads to fluid retention – which is the last thing you need when you are having a period.*

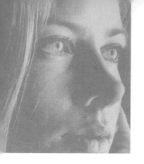

# Premenstrual syndrome: PMS

*Recurrent symptoms may include back ache, headache, bloated abdomen, cramps, breast tenderness, irrational behaviour, anxiety, depression and poor concentration.*

**P**remenstrual syndrome is the most common of all menstrual problems *(see p.106)* and around 70 per cent of women who are still having a menstrual cycle will suffer from it to some extent. The physical and mental changes may begin just after mid-cycle, but usually occur in the seven days preceding menstruation and vanish as soon as the period starts. Sadly, PMS is still a much under-rated problem, from a medical standpoint, but even in mild cases it can be distressing.

START OF PERIOD

PMS SYMPTOMS

MID-CYCLE OVULATION

**ABOVE** Monitoring your menstrual cycle enables you to become familiar with potential problems and take remedial steps accordingly.

🌑 **Call the doctor**
*If your symptoms are significantly interfering with your life.*

## ✚ CONVENTIONAL MEDICINE

Keep a chart showing when symptoms occur in relation to menstruation, to enable you to rearrange schedules to avoid particularly difficult days and help to determine whether remedies are of benefit. Breast pain may be helped by products that contain gamolenic acid (otherwise known as evening primrose oil). If premenstrual syndrome is severe, your doctor may recommend hormonal treatments and possibly even counselling.

DOSAGE: ADULTS AND CHILDREN OVER 16  3–4 capsules of gamolenic acid twice a day, usually for 2–3 months; consult pack for details.

## HERBAL REMEDIES

Agnus-castus is often effective for PMS.
USE AND DOSAGE  Take 10–20 drops of tincture each morning, increasing to 20–40 drops in the 10 days before the period is due.

Helonias, an ovarian stimulant, is available in capsules and tablets, and Dang Gui is also becoming more readily obtainable.

You can make a simple herbal tea from equal amounts of St John's wort, raspberry leaf and vervain for daily use.

## ✿ HOMEOPATHIC REMEDIES

A prescription based on the individual is usually most successful, so consult a qualified homeopath.

**Lilium tigrinum 30c**

For snappy, irritable person. Worse for sympathy. Must keep busy. Heavy period pains, uterus feels as though congested.

**Pulsatilla 30c**

For weepy person, who feels unloved and wants sympathy. PMS starts at puberty. Changeable in mood and symptom. Chilly, but dislikes stuffy room. **DOSAGE** I tablet twice daily until improved. Maximum I week. May be repeated at the next period.

**ABOVE** Oysters are an excellent source of zinc, which plays a role in regulating PMS.

## AROMATHERAPY

- Geranium *(Pelargonium graveolens)*
- Fennel *(Foeniculum vulgare)*
- Clary sage *(Salvia sclarea)*
- Rose *(Rosa damascena/Rosa centifolia)*
- Ylang ylang *(Cananga odorata)*
- Neroli *(Citrus aurantium)*
- Sandalwood *(Santalum album)*
- Vetivert *(Vetiveria zizanoides)*
- Jasmine *(Jasminum officinale)*
- Bergamot *(Citrus bergamia)*

You will have to decide, by trial and error, which of these oils best suits your own range of symptoms. **APPLICATION** Use in a way that suits your condition.

YLANG YLANG

## NUTRITION

It is not just what you eat that is important, but what you *don't* eat and *when* you eat. Women with PMS should eat little and often (never going more than 2 hours without food) and include plenty of complex carbohydrates (wholemeal bread, rice, pasta, potatoes, root vegetables, beans) with sensible protein like fish, eggs, cheese, poultry and lean meat. Sweet cravings can be satisfied by fruit. Eat plenty of dark green leafy vegetables and wholemeal bread; extra-virgin olive oil, nuts and seeds; shellfish, oysters and pumpkin seeds. Avoid consuming excessive salt, caffeine and alcohol.

CAMOMILE

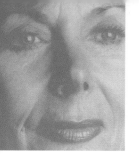

# Menopause

*No periods for more than one year; sudden attacks of hot flushes; dry vagina, sometimes causing pain during intercourse; urinary problems, including incontinence; may be associated with depression and anxiety.*

**S**ome women sail through the menopause; for others it represents months, and sometimes years, of misery. But the menopause is not a disease; it is in fact, for many women, the beginning of years free from the monthly discomfort of difficult periods and contraception. Home remedies can strengthen the bones, protect against heart disease and keep your skin healthy. Anorexia, overexercising and simply being too thin can all affect hormone production and cause an artificial menopause. Having both ovaries removed has the same result.

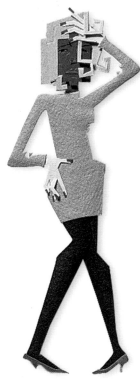

**ABOVE** Symptoms of the menopause can be controlled to let you lead a full and active life.

### ✚ CONVENTIONAL MEDICINE

Hormone replacement therapy (HRT) can help to alleviate difficult symptoms and to reduce the risk of osteoporosis and heart disease in later life. It is given in the form of tablets, patches, gels or cream, and may cause a regular bleed. Consult your doctor for further details.

### ▨ HERBAL REMEDIES

Night sweats, hot flushes and palpitations may be eased by herbal remedies.

USE AND DOSAGE Make up equal amounts of vervain, sage, mugwort and motherwort (2tsp per cup) as a tea. Sage is rich in hormonal compounds, so a regular daily cup can be helpful.

The Chinese herbal tonic for this time is He Shou Wu (also called Fo Ti), now available in many health-food stores.

### ◖ AROMATHERAPY

- 🌿 Geranium *(Pelargonium graveolens)*
- 🌿 Rose *(Rosa damascena/Rosa centifolia)*
- 🌿 Fennel *(Foeniculum vulgare)*

Geranium helps to balance the hormones; fennel produces a plant oestrogen; and rose regulates the menstrual cycle. Also try any of the antidepressant oils or those for symptomatic conditions, such as constipation (see p.96).

**APPLICATION** Use in baths, in creams or in foot spas – whatever method is most convenient for you. Supplementation with starflower may also help.

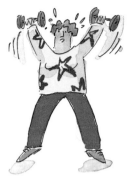

## HOMEOPATHIC REMEDIES

Homeopathy can be used to treat the symptoms of the menopause.

### ∽ Lachesis 30c

For person who may be talkative, jealous, worse for any sleep or alcohol. Palpitations and flushes. Probably the remedy used most often.

### ∽ Sepia 30c

For lack of emotions, indifference to own family, loss of sex drive. Weeping and feelings of guilt. Flushes with fainting. Better for being alone.

**DOSAGE** 1 tablet twice daily. Maximum 1 week.

## NUTRITION

Good nutrition is the easiest way to reduce the risk of post-menopausal complications, especially if you decide not to take HRT. Plan your daily eating to include the specific nutrients your body now needs in greater abundance than ever: calcium and vitamin D to protect your bones – so eat plenty of low-fat dairy products, sardines and other oily fish (with their bones when possible), dark green leafy vegetables and chickpeas; vitamins A, C and E, lots of beta-carotene, soluble fibre and essential fatty acids – so eat avocados, olive oil, nuts and seeds, oats, brown rice, wholegrain cereals, apricots, carrots and broccoli, liver at least once a week and lots of oily fish; copious quantities of cabbage and its relatives. You should also eat soya bean products often.

This is one time in your life when regular vitamin and mineral supplements can be a real bonus: a daily multivitamin and mineral supplement, a calcium with vitamin D supplement and 1g of evening primrose oil. To help with hot flushes, a combination of vitamin $B_6$, magnesium and zinc can be added.

**BELOW** Curly kale is full of vitamin D, essential for strong bones.

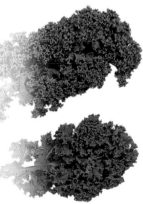

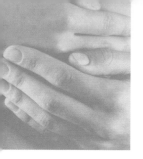

# Thrush: Candida

*Symptoms are a thick, creamy-white vaginal discharge; sore, itchy vagina, with discomfort along the lips of the vagina; painful intercourse; and a burning sensation when passing urine.*

Thrush is a common infection that is caused by the yeast organism *Candida albicans*. 'Thrush' usually means vaginal infection, however, as opposed to the other common sites of *Candida* infection, which are in the mouth and throat and around the anus or areas of damaged skin. Vaginal thrush may be accompanied by pain and burning when passing urine, together with a thick discharge and severe itching and discomfort along the lips of the vagina. For many years the home remedies of complementary practitioners have offered effective treatment.

### ✚ CONVENTIONAL MEDICINE

Conventional treatment is usually with antifungal medicines, which can be inserted into the vagina as pessaries or taken by mouth as a single tablet. When a woman has recurrent thrush infections, her partner may need treatment.

DOSAGE: ADULTS  A single large-dose pessary can be used, although smaller doses taken over consecutive days may be preferred; follow medical advice. Or a single tablet can be taken by mouth. All treatment may be combined with an antifungal cream for external use.

**BELOW** Lemon balm is anti-fungal and can be beneficial for those suffering from thrush.

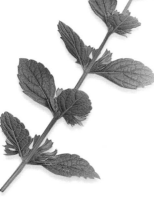

### HERBAL REMEDIES

Antifungal and antiseptic herbs – such as echinacea, garlic, camomile, lemon balm, thyme and marigold – as well as immune stimulants like astragalus and reishi can all help candidiasis. The Amazonian herb pau d'arco is popular and available in tablet form.

USE AND DOSAGE  Try an infusion of marigold, lemon balm, camomile and elderflowers (2tsp per cup, four times daily).

For vaginal thrush, try tea-tree or thyme oil pessaries, or put 2 drops of tea-tree oil onto a moistened tampon, insert and leave for up to 4 hours.

## ✿ HOMEOPATHIC REMEDIES

A consultation with a homeopath is recommended.

**Borax 6c**

For itchy vulva. Discharge thick or like white of egg, makes vulva sore. Discharge before and after period.

**Helonias 6c**

For creamy-white discharge, which may recur with itching and soreness of vulva.

DOSAGE 1 tablet twice daily. Maximum 2 weeks.

**Candida albicans 30c**

For recurrent thrush.

DOSAGE 1 tablet 12-hourly. Maximum three doses.

## AROMATHERAPY

**Lavender** *(Lavandula angustifolia)*

**Tea tree** *(Melaleuca alternifolia)*

**Myrrh** *(Commiphora molmol)*

**Palmarosa** *(Cymbopogon martinii)*

Lavender eases the pain and promotes healing. Tea tree and myrrh act against the organism that causes thrush (but use tea tree in a low dilution, as it can irritate the mucous membrane). Palmarosa helps to balance intestinal flora. Treatment needs to be long-term or thrush may recur.

APPLICATION Use in the bath or as a compress on the outer areas. Palmarosa can also be used as a massage oil for the abdominal area.

## NUTRITION

Garlic is a powerful antifungal and should be used generously – at least two whole cloves a day, added to recipes or just eaten in a sandwich, are essential. It also helps to eat a good portion of live yogurt daily, to maintain the balance of beneficial probiotic bacteria in the gut, which may help to prevent the spread of the *Candida* infection. All the B vitamins are important too, so eat plenty of complex carbohydrates, like wholemeal bread, pasta and brown rice; and eat extra muesli, sunflower seeds, lentils and white fish for their rich vitamin $B_6$ content.

Get extra zinc from eggs, sardines, oysters, most other shellfish and pumpkin seeds.

### Prevention

*It is best to avoid wearing synthetic knickers, and tights should have a cotton gusset – or, better still, wear stockings. Avoid very hot baths, antiseptic soaps, excessive washing and all highly perfumed, foaming bath additives.*

*Some complementary practitioners advise extreme yeast-excluding diets, but there is no scientific basis for these. It is advisable, however, to reduce your sugar consumption, as a high sugar intake can encourage the growth of Candida.*

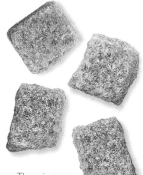

**ABOVE** There is some evidence that reducing your sugar intake can lower the risk of thrush.

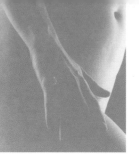

CRAMP
BARK

# Fibroids

*Most women have no symptoms, but there may be heavy
menstrual bleeding; an urge to pass urine frequently, caused
by the fibroids pressing on surrounding organs, such as the
bladder; the lower part of the abdomen may swell.*

These benign tumours develop in the smooth muscle of the uterus
and around 20 per cent of women over the age of 35 will be
affected. They are more common in Afro-Caribbean women. They are
probably the most common reason for a hysterectomy, but less invasive
medical techniques can now be used and self-help may contain their
growth until the menopause. After this time the decline in the body's
production of oestrogen results in a gradual reduction in fibroid size.

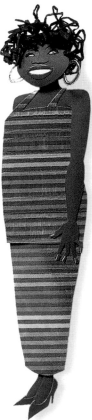

**BELOW** Women with
fibroids may benefit
from drinking simple
herbal infusions.

### ✚ CONVENTIONAL MEDICINE

Most fibroids do not need any treatment, but if
symptoms are troublesome, seek medical advice. If
medicines are unsuccessful, surgery may remove
the fibroids or the whole womb (hysterectomy).

### HERBAL REMEDIES

Treatment should really be left to professionals,
although simple remedies can ease symptoms.
**USE AND DOSAGE** Cramp bark or black haw, in
decoction or tinctures, eases pain. Shepherd's purse
infusion (1tsp per cup) can help stop bleeding. Or
make a tea of violet leaves, shepherd's purse and
motherwort (2tsp per cup, drunk three times a day).

### ❁ HOMEOPATHIC REMEDIES

It is best to consult a qualified homeopath. The
following remedies may be a guide.

⌒ **Ustilago 6c**
For left-sided ovarian pain, which may extend to
the legs. Fibroids with heavy periods and clots,
especially when approaching the menopause.

⌒ **Fraxinus americana 6c**
For fibroids with heavy feeling in vagina. Watery
vaginal discharge.
**DOSAGE** 1 tablet daily. Maximum 2 weeks.

# The Excretory System

The kidneys filter about 150l/300pt of fluid each day, producing about 900ml/1½pt of urine and returning the rest to the circulation. If the bladder or urethra becomes infected, cystitis may result; bedwetting, on the other hand, may occur for no apparent reason and is usually self-limiting in children. Piles or haemorrhoids are another uncomfortable disorder of the excretory system. But relief for all these ailments is at hand, using simple nutritional, aromatherapeutic, herbal and homeopathic remedies, supported by conventional treatment.

# Haemorrhoids

*Characterized by bleeding, often a bright red streak on the toilet paper or surface of the faeces; part of the bowel may prolapse (stick out) when faeces are passed, then may return or stay out.*

If you have had children, suffer from constipation, stand a lot at work or are seriously overweight, the chances are that you will suffer from haemorrhoids (or piles, as they are more colloquially known) at some point. If severe, haemorrhoids – which are varicose veins in the soft lining of the anus – may require surgical treatment, but home remedies can provide great relief for most people.

## ⚫ Call the doctor

*If you have had any bleeding from the anus, in order to rule out a more serious cause.*

### ✚ CONVENTIONAL MEDICINE

Eat plenty of high-fibre foods, such as apples, pears, beans, oats, wholemeal bread and brown rice. Drink plenty of water. This will help to keep the faeces soft and avoid straining to pass a bowel motion. Your doctor may prescribe suppositories together with cream containing anti-inflammatory drugs.

### HERBAL REMEDIES

One traditional – but effective – herb for haemorrhoids is pilewort, so called in the Middle Ages because its roots actually resemble piles. It is extremely astringent and heals the damaged tissues. USE AND DOSAGE Ointments made from both pilewort leaves and root are readily available, or the dried herb can be taken internally in capsules.

Infusions of yarrow, lime flowers or melilot will help the circulation and blood vessels, while fresh *Aloe vera* leaves, distilled witch hazel, chickweed cream or borage juice can relieve itching.

### ✤ HOMEOPATHIC REMEDIES

Unexplained or persistent rectal bleeding requires medical attention. Paeonia ointment may help to relieve the itching.

⬧ Aesculus 6c

For sensation of splinters felt in rectum. Pain

extends to hips. Large, painful and protruding, purple haemorrhoids. Anus is dry and itchy.

**Aloe 6c**

For piles like bunches of grapes. Purple colour, better for cold bathing. Itching in rectum. Diarrhoea.

**Hamamelis 6c**

For haemorrhoids in pregnancy, profuse bleeding with soreness.

*Dosage:* 1 tablet twice daily. Maximum 2 weeks.

## AROMATHERAPY

**Cypress** *(Cupressus sempervirens)*
**Geranium** *(Pelargonium graveolens)*
**Juniper** *(Juniperus communis)*
**Myrrh** *(Commiphora molmol)*

These oils help to increase the circulation. Cypress is a natural astringent, which can help shrink the piles. **APPLICATION** Use either alternate hot and cold sitz baths or 3–4 drops of your chosen oil in a warm compress, held on the anus or against the haemorrhoid. Or add about 10 drops of geranium and 10 drops of cypress to a whole tube of lubrication jelly, mix together and apply; store in a small jar.

**ABOVE** Relieve the discomfort by applying aromatherapy oils either as a bath or as a compress.

## NUTRITION

During an episode of painful haemorrhoids it is important to keep the stool as soft as possible. Dried fruit, especially prunes and apricots, and a regular intake of prune juice will help. Avoid the temptation not to pass stools, however painful it might be, as further constipation will only make the piles worse. Plenty of fluid and foods rich in soluble fibre, such as oats, apples, pears and nearly all vegetables, will help prevent constipation leading to haemorrhoids. If you are constantly losing even small amounts of blood from your piles there is a risk of anaemia, so take nutritional steps to prevent this *(see p.56).* This is particularly important for women, especially during pregnancy.

Avoid food with lots of seeds (e.g. tomatoes, raspberries) until your condition has settled down, because these can cause further irritation.

### Caution

Do not apply the essential oils neat. If there is any bleeding, seek medical advice before using essential oils.

### Prevention

To prevent haemorrhoids it is important to stimulate blood flow to the rectum area. The best way to do this is by daily contrast bathing with alternate hot and cold water.

# Cystitis

*Painful, burning sensation when passing urine, often worse at end of stream; urine may be pink, due to the presence of blood; there may be small blood clots; frequent need to go to the toilet, perhaps only passing a small amount; fever.*

**C**ystitis can be an isolated acute problem or a recurring chronic nightmare, which affects millions of women but few men. It is often impossible to trace the specific bacteria that trigger an episode of cystitis, which is often linked to concurrent attacks of thrush *(see p.112)*. Recurrent episodes may be treated with prophylactic antibiotics.

## 🌐 Call the doctor

*If you have a high fever with cystitis and/or vomiting; if you have cystitis with back pain; if your symptoms persist.*

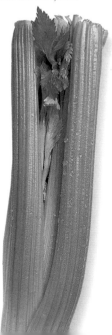

**BELOW** Celery and other diuretic foods will help flush out the system.

## ✚ CONVENTIONAL MEDICINE

Over-the-counter remedies help neutralize the acid in the urine. If symptoms remain, antibiotics are usually required to prevent the infection spreading to the kidneys.

**DOSAGE: ADULTS** Take antibiotics up to three or four times a day for 3–7 days; follow medical advice.

**DOSAGE: CHILDREN** Give antibiotic syrup up to four times a day. Dose depends on age and weight of the child; follow medical advice and remember to complete the course.

## 🍎 NUTRITION

Drink at least 2.25–2.75l/4–5pt of water each day and make sure you eat plenty of the diuretic foods, such as celery, parsley and dandelion leaves. Avoid caffeine, drink little alcohol and only weak tea.

The traditional kitchen treatment for cystitis is lemon barley water. Pour 900ml/1½pt of boiling water over 50g/2oz of washed barley and the grated rind and juice of an unwaxed lemon. Add ½tsp of sugar, stir thoroughly and drink one glass three times a day. Modern scientific research, however, has now proved that a traditional Native North American remedy – cranberry juice – is even more effective. Chemicals in the juice seem to prevent the cystitis-causing bacteria from making their home in the bladder tissue. Drink at least

600ml/1pt a day of a 50:50 dilution of cranberry juice with water. This acts both as treatment during an attack of cystitis and as long-term protection.

### HERBAL REMEDIES

Many herbs act as urinary antiseptics and can be helpful in combating infections and inflammation, while drinking herbal teas provides a necessary increase in fluid intake.

USE AND DOSAGE Take up to 4 cups daily of a tea made from 1 part each of buchu, couchgrass, bearberry and cornsilk (2tsp per cup of water). Add 2 parts shepherd's purse if there is blood in the urine, but make sure that you seek professional advice if symptoms persist.

Avoid spicy foods and those producing acid residues, such as meat and shellfish.

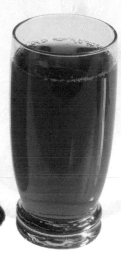

ABOVE Cranberry juice and lemon barley water are effective in the treatment and prevention of cystitis.

### AROMATHERAPY

- Myrrh (*Commiphora molmol*)
- Tea tree (*Melaleuca alternifolia*)
- Roman camomile (*Chamaemelum nobile*)
- Lavender (*Lavandula angustifolia*)

These oils are calming, soothing and anti-inflammatory; tea tree is antiviral, antifungal and antibacterial.

APPLICATION Use in a warm compress over the lower back, in sitz baths or in ordinary baths.

### HOMEOPATHIC REMEDIES

Symptoms in males or worsening symptoms, back pain or chills require medical help.

- Cantharis 30c

For 'peeing red hot needles'. Constantly wanting to urinate, but passing just a few drops. Urine may be bloody.

- Staphysagria 30c

For 'honeymoon cystitis'. Burning pain after intercourse or after having had a catheter inserted. Recurrent cystitis related to intercourse.

DOSAGE 1 tablet every 4 hours until condition improves. Maximum 5 days.

**Caution**

*If blood or pus appears in the urine, contact your doctor immediately. If antibiotics are prescribed, continue with the aromatherapy treatment, as they will work side-by-side.*

# Bedwetting: enuresis

*Uncontrollable urge to pass urine in a child who is learning to use a toilet; adults may also suffer, particularly after undergoing an alcoholic binge.*

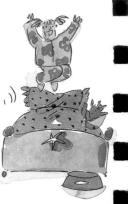

**B**edwetting is much more common in boys than girls, and most children grow out of it by the age of four or five. It is seldom the result of underlying disease, although occasionally it may be. It can be the result of stress, anxiety or other behavioural disturbances, but in most instances 'just happens'.

🌐 **Call the doctor**

*If bedwetting does not improve after trying these remedies.*

**BELOW** With very young children, patience and understanding might be the only treatment that is needed.

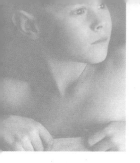

## ✚ CONVENTIONAL MEDICINE

There is no fixed age at which a child should be dry at night, but bedwetting from the age of seven is often treated by doctors. A child who has been dry might wet the bed when starting a new school, or because of a urine infection. Avoid scolding or withholding drinks – encouragement to use the toilet is more effective. Reward a dry night with approval.

## HERBAL REMEDIES

During the day, give dilute herbal teas to help strengthen the bladder and soothe distress.

**USE AND DOSAGE** Mix 1tsp each of cornsilk, shepherd's purse and skullcap and infuse in 250ml/8fl oz of water. Give children under three half a cup, with 1tsp of pasteurized honey, two to three times daily. One hour before bedtime give 10 drops of sweet sumach tincture, diluted in 5ml/1tsp of water.

## ❋ HOMEOPATHIC REMEDIES

🌿 **Causticum 6c**

For sensitive person, who wets bed during early part of sleep or in daytime when sneezing/coughing.

🌿 **Equisetum 6c**

For person who has dreams/nightmares when passing urine. Bedwetting in children and elderly women.

**DOSAGE** 1 tablet before bed. Maximum 2 weeks.

# The Senses

The largest organ of our bodies, skin is a remarkable substance, acting as a protective barrier for all the internal body organs, eliminating waste products through sweat and being ultra-sensitive to pain, touch and temperature. But it is also subject to numerous disorders, from acne and warts to dermatitis and cellulite, and needs nourishment in order to remain healthy. Other senses – such as hearing, sight and taste – manifest problems in the form of complaints such as earache, conjunctivitis and mouth ulcers. But relief is available through both internal and external remedies.

# Acne

*Characterized by blackheads, spots and greasy skin, most frequently appearing on the face, but also sometimes erupting on the neck, shoulders, back or chest; most common among teenagers.*

**A**cne is a distressing skin problem that affects around 80 per cent of young people between the ages of 12 and 24. It occurs as a result of a build-up of oil or sebum secreted through the pores, which become blocked, then infected, causing spots. It is more common in boys than girls and is triggered by the fluctuating levels of hormones during adolescence. Diet can play a vital part in improving, or worsening, acne.

**BELOW** Teenagers should eat a diet high in fruit and vegetables to keep their system as free as possible from the toxins that encourage acne.

## CONVENTIONAL MEDICINE

Mild acne may only require a lotion that dries the skin. In moderately severe cases, an antibiotic preparation applied to the skin may be used in combination with a drying lotion. If acne is persistent, antibiotic tablets may be more effective. In severe cases, treatment with a derivative of vitamin A may be prescribed by a dermatologist. Most treatments take up to 3–6 months to work and may need to be continued beyond this.

DOSAGE: ADULTS AND CHILDREN   Apply lotions and creams to the whole area, not just the spots, twice a day. Tablets may be taken once a day or more often; follow medical advice.

## HERBAL REMEDIES

Combine cleansing herbs taken internally with external antiseptic washes, steam baths or lotions. USE AND DOSAGE   Drink 3 cups daily of a tea made by infusing 10g/¼oz each of agrimony, burdock leaves and marigold petals in 500ml/18fl oz of water.

Apply a lotion of 50ml/2fl oz each of distilled witch hazel and rosewater with 5ml/1tsp each of tea-tree and thyme oils.

You can also rub acne pustules with a garlic clove each night.

## AROMATHERAPY

- Lavender *(Lavandula angustifolia)*
- Bergamot *(Citrus bergamia)*
- Tea tree *(Melaleuca alternifolia)*

These oils are bactericidal and relaxing, which will help with stress. Tea tree builds up the body's immune system.

**APPLICATION** Apply lavender neat, using a cotton bud, directly to the spot. All three oils can be used in a compress or facial steamer; and in a bath.

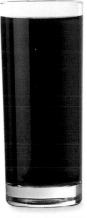

**ABOVE** Sweet, fizzy drinks and chocolate should be avoided if a clear skin is to be maintained.

## NUTRITION

Avoid high-fat, high-sugar convenience foods; eliminate chocolate, ice cream, salt, burgers and all manufactured meat products. A detox programme of raw fruit, vegetables and salads with unlimited water, unsalted vegetable juices and herbal teas should be followed for 3 days each month. After the third day add wholegrains and cooked vegetables, returning to your normal diet on the fourth day.

Eat plenty of dark green and orange vegetables and fruit for their beta-carotene; citrus fruit for their vitamin C; tropical fruit for their high enzyme content; nuts, seeds and vegetable oils for their vitamin E. Eat some cabbage every day. Complex carbohydrates, like potatoes, brown rice and wholemeal bread, can be eaten in abundance. Use vegetarian protein sources or fish and lean poultry.

> **Caution**
> Do not apply any oil other than lavender directly to the skin.

KIWI FRUIT

## HOMEOPATHIC REMEDIES

A consultation with a homeopath is recommended.
- Kali bromatum 6c

For acne of face, cheek and forehead. Spots look bluish-red, discharge pus and produce scars.
- Sulphur 6c

For spots on forehead and nose. Skin worse for washing, sensitive to cold air. Spots that are scratched discharge pus. Patient intolerant of heat, lazy and produces smelly sweat.

**DOSAGE** 1 tablet daily. Maximum 2 weeks.

# Boils

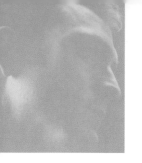

*An infection that starts around a hair follicle, forming pus, with localized swelling; hot, red skin over the affected area; pain, often throbbing, sometimes associated with a yellow discharge of pus.*

**A**nyone can get a boil at any time, and the occasional episode is painful and unpleasant, but not of great significance, as long as it is treated correctly. Repeated boils may, however, be a sign of underlying illness (for example, diabetes) or an indication that your natural resistance has declined for some reason. The most likely sites for boils to erupt are at the back of the neck, on the nostrils, armpits and between the legs and buttocks.

**BELOW** A boil is unsightly and depressing, but it seldom has any long-term effects.

## CONVENTIONAL MEDICINE

A boil may burst spontaneously or it may need lancing in order to release the pus. Treatment at an early stage with antibiotics can sometimes prevent a boil from developing, as can cleaning all cuts well with soap and water.

**DOSAGE: ADULTS** Take antibiotics three or four times a day for a period of 3–7 days; follow medical advice.

**DOSAGE: CHILDREN** Give antibiotic syrup up to four times a day; take medical advice.

## HERBAL REMEDIES

Traditionally herbalists use poultices or drawing ointments in order to encourage boils to discharge. You can apply commercially available slippery elm or chickweed ointments, or make yourself a slippery elm poultice

**USE AND DOSAGE** Mix 1tsp of powdered slippery elm with enough hot water, or hot marigold infusion, to make a thick paste, then apply to the boil. Apply a little echinacea or marigold cream to clear any remaining infection.

Internally, garlic or echinacea (2 x 200mg capsules, twice a day) will help improve resistance to further infection.

## AROMATHERAPY

- Tea tree *(Melaleuca alternifolia)*
- Lavender *(Lavandula angustifolia)*
- Bergamot *(Citrus bergamia)*
- Juniper *(Juniperus communis)*

Tea tree is bactericidal. Lavender is calming, soothing and a natural painkiller, as is bergamot. Juniper helps to detoxify the system.

APPLICATION Use tea tree, lavender and bergamot in a hot compress; juniper and lavender in the bath.

## HOMEOPATHIC REMEDIES

- Belladonna 6c

For sudden onset, skin painful, red, hot and throbbing. First stages of boil with little pus formation.

- Hepar sulphuris calcareum 6c

For splinter-like pains at slightest touch. Brings boil to a head. Patient may be bad-tempered.

- Sulphur 6c

For crops of boils in different places on the body. One boil finishes as another starts.

DOSAGE 1 tablet every 4 hours for 2–3 days or until improved.

## NUTRITION

Eat plenty of vitamin C-rich food – blackcurrants, blueberries, citrus fruit, kiwis and fresh fruit juices; liver, carrots, broccoli and spinach for their vitamin A; pumpkin seeds and shellfish for their zinc; garlic and cabbage for their anti-bacterial properties. Avoiding high-sugar and high-fat foods substantially reduces the risk of getting boils, so eat less sugar and refined carbohydrates and drink fewer sweetened fizzy drinks.

**Prevention**
*A healthy diet (see Nutrition) based on plenty of fresh fruit and vegetables and a low sugar intake, is the best way to avoid getting boils.*

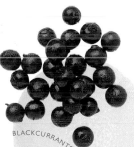

**BELOW** Blackcurrants, garlic, broccoli, citrus fruit, pumpkin seeds and shellfish all contain beneficial nutrients.

BLACKCURRANTS

GARLIC

BROCCOLI

# Warts

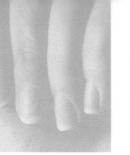

*An unsightly skin growth, often having no symptoms, although they may cause pain if found on the sole of the foot.*

MARIGOLD

**W**arts are caused by the human papilloma virus and they are generally spread from another part of the body or caught from someone else. Most people with warts will lose them as the wart virus dies off. For the remainder, they can vary from a mildly irritating single wart to painful plantar warts, or verrucae, and large, conjoined groups of distressing genital warts, which may also put these women's babies at risk. Genital warts can be sexually transmitted and both partners should ensure that they receive medical attention.

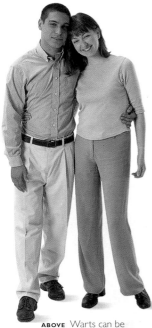

**ABOVE** Warts can be passed from person to person so they should be treated, even though they generally cause no discomfort.

## ✚ CONVENTIONAL MEDICINE

Most warts will disappear eventually with no treatment, but because they can spread or be painful, many people opt to treat them.

The principle of all treatment for warts is to try and destroy the wart tissue without actually harming the surrounding normal skin. Keep the wart covered to avoid spreading the infection. Before applying a treatment, file the surface of the wart to remove any hard skin, but make sure that the skin is not open or cracked. Seek medical advice for persistent or spreading warts.

DOSAGE: ADULTS AND CHILDREN  Apply the treatment daily after filing the surface with an emery board or pumice stone; consult pack for details.

## HERBAL REMEDIES

Thuja is extremely antiviral and antifungal.

USE AND DOSAGE  A couple of drops of tincture on the wart night and morning will usually clear it reasonably quickly. Also take 5 drops of tincture in a little water twice a day.

Other useful herbs include tea-tree oil, marigold, *Aloe vera*, house leeks and the sap of freshly picked greater celandine.

## AROMATHERAPY

- Lemon *(Citrus limon)*
- Tea tree *(Melaleuca alternifolia)*

Tea tree is antiviral, while both lemon and tea-tree oil are antiseptic.

**APPLICATION** Apply neat essential oil using a toothpick, so that you get 1 drop directly onto the wart or verruca. Cover with a dry plaster or dressing and repeat at least twice a day. Alternate the lemon and tea-tree oils after 2 or 3 weeks for maximum effect.

## HOMEOPATHIC REMEDIES

- Thuja 6c

For large, jagged, cauliflower warts. Large, flat warts located on the hands and fingers. Nails deformed. Painful verrucae. This is probably the most common remedy for warts.

- Causticum 6c

For warts situated on hands, face and lips. Bleed easily. Warts inflamed and hard; located near or under fingernails.

- Nitric acid 6c

For large, soft, yellow warts. Especially on eyelids and nose. Bleed on washing. Soft warts.

- Dulcamara 6c

For smooth, large warts on face or palm.

**DOSAGE** 1 tablet taken twice daily until improved. Maximum 3 weeks.

## NUTRITION

Diet itself cannot really help in treating warts, but foodstuffs have traditionally been used: simple, non-genital warts may respond to rubbing them with the cut end of a clove of garlic, a cut dandelion stalk or even undiluted lemon juice. Repeat twice daily for a week or two. And if you have a fig tree in your garden, a milky latex can be squeezed from the leaf or stem and dropped onto the wart. Wear rubber gloves and cover the adjacent skin with petroleum jelly. After a few hours an inflamed ring of skin will surround the wart, which should soon shrivel up and drop off. Repeat after a few days, if necessary.

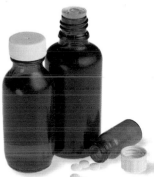

**BELOW** Treatment with aromatherapy or homeopathic remedies takes several weeks, but is usually effective.

# Corns and calluses

*An area of thick, hardened skin, which may be painful;*
*often found on the toes, although it may also manifest itself*
*on the hands after rough, repetitive manual work such*
*as gardening.*

orns and calluses of the feet are the inevitable result of wearing ill-fitting shoes. If there are deformities of the foot, these can also lead to areas of excessive pressure or a change of weight distribution when standing or walking. Either way, corns or calluses may result. Corns should be dealt with by a qualified chiropodist and should not be hacked at with any of the patent corn-removing gadgets. Calluses may also occur on the palms of the hand and the fingers – for example, as the result of gardening or manual work.

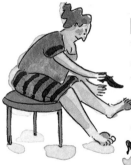

### ✚ CONVENTIONAL MEDICINE

You can gently file a callus and then moisturize the skin. It may be easier to file the skin after a bath, when the skin is soft and pliable.

Covering a corn with a cushioned plaster, which is designed to avoid putting pressure directly on the corn itself, can help to relieve the pain. Otherwise, seek professional advice from a qualified podiatrist.

### ✿ HOMEOPATHIC REMEDIES

There are various homeopathic treatments that may help alleviate corns and calluses.

**Antimonium crudum 6c**
For thick and distorted nails. Horny lumps on hands and soles. Callosities from slight pressure. Inflamed corns. Feet very tender.

**Graphites 6c**
For thick, ingrown and crumbling nails. Callosities on the hands, with skin that cracks and discharges sticky substance.

**Ferrum picricum 6c**
For corns with yellowish discoloration. May also be many warts on the hands.

**DOSAGE:** 1 tablet twice daily. Maximum 2 weeks.

## Prevention

*Shoes should have a round rather than pointed shape, and there should be at least 2.5cm/1in between the end of the longest toe and the tip of the inside of the shoe. Avoid high-heeled and court shoes, which cram the foot down into the toe end.*

**ABOVE** Any of these culinary items can be used to treat corns, but professional advice should be sought if the corns do not improve.

### HERBAL REMEDIES

There are numerous traditional herbal remedies for corns, such as mashed house leeks, onions, garlic cloves or lemon rind and juice applied directly to the affected area. Inflammation can be soothed with St John's wort cream or comfrey oil, while easing pressure on the area with thick felt rings. Rubbing the feet with fresh plantain leaves was traditionally believed to prevent corns.

### Caution

Do not use corn removing gadgets; instead, seek advice from a qualified podiatrist or chiropodist.

### AROMATHERAPY

- Roman camomile *(Chamaemelum nobile)*
- Lavender *(Lavandula angustifolia)*
- Good-quality vegetable oil (or calendula oil: available from reputable suppliers)

Roman camomile and lavender are both anti-inflammatory, so they will bring the swelling down and thus lessen the pain of corns and calluses. Using a good-quality vegetable oil will reduce the areas of hard skin.

**APPLICATION** Use in a daily massage, especially combining the essential oil with the good quality vegetable oil. If there is inflammation and the affected area is too tender to touch, then foot baths (or hand baths, if the calluses are on the hand) will be more relevant.

ST JOHN'S WORT

# Cellulite

*Pitted orange-peel appearance on the skin, most frequently occurring on the upper thighs, buttocks and arms, where women have a higher proportion of fat than men; primarily a female condition.*

This much-discussed and written about 'ailment' is not an illness at all. The orange-peel-like skin that characterizes cellulite is not the result of a build-up of toxins, but rather something that happens to the skin of most women – and 98 per cent of cellulite sufferers are female. This is because women have a thinner outer skin than men, a thinner underlying level of the dermis and a different composition of fat cells in the subcutaneous layer. Cellulite is caused by a combination of hormone changes, skin structure and fat deposits, and though it occurs in women of all sizes, it is more common in those who are overweight.

**BELOW** A sensible diet is likely to be more effective in reducing cellulite than expensive creams.

## ✚ CONVENTIONAL MEDICINE

Cellulite may improve by taking regular exercise and shedding excess weight, although it tends to worsen during pregnancy. There is no evidence to suggest that rubbing in expensive moisturizers and oils has any positive effect.

## NUTRITION

Despite being a cosmetic problem, cellulite is the cause of considerable distress to those suffering from it and, since a woman's total number of fat cells is partially determined by her mother's nutrition during pregnancy, there are certain women who are more prone to it than others.

Weight loss is the first step towards the reduction of cellulite, but do take care: if you lose weight too quickly the condition gets worse. So no crash diets, no ridiculous regimes of meal replacements and pills, just sensible eating (see *Weight Problems* on p.100), together with a reduction of refined carbohydrates – from sugars, biscuits, cakes, sweets and fizzy drinks. A diet that is high in complex carbohydrates (such as wholemeal cereals, pasta, beans, potatoes) will ensure that you get an adequate intake of both soluble and insoluble fibre. This in turns helps remove cholesterol from the body and keep fat out of the diet. So eat plenty of brown rice, oats, beans, wholemeal bread and pasta for their fibre; sweet peppers, broccoli, spinach and sweet potatoes for their beta-carotene; small amounts of liver for its vitamin A, an essential nutrient for skin health. Reduce your intake of salt and cut down on alcohol, both of which interfere with the efficient circulation of blood to the skin.

> **Caution**
> *Rosemary and fennel oils must not be used by those with high blood pressure or epilepsy.*

### AROMATHERAPY

- Juniper *(Juniperus communis)*
- Fennel *(Foeniculum vulgare)*
- Rosemary *(Rosmarinus officinalis)*

Fennel is a diuretic. Juniper will help the body to detoxify and rosemary helps to stimulate the lymphatic system, which enables the body to remove waste products. If a hormone imbalance is suspected, then geranium (which is another diuretic) could also be used.

APPLICATION Use these oils as a massage and in baths (including foot baths). You are looking for long-term benefits, as there is no short term relief. The skin will feel better before it actually looks better. Remember that stress can be a factor (see p.36).

JUNIPER BERRIES

### HERBAL REMEDIES

Popular demand has created a variety of over-the-counter herbal products purporting to reduce cellulite. Most are based on metabolic stimulants, such as kelp, to encourage weight loss and should not be used for more than 2–3 weeks. Avoid over-the-counter cellulite remedies based on powerful laxatives (for example, senna, cascara sagrada, rhubarb root), designed to cause sudden weight loss. Patent skin rubs are often based on rubefacient oils, such as juniper or pepper, which increase surface blood flow in an attempt to revive tired tissues.

# Dermatitis

*Starts as a patch of itchy skin covered with small blisters, often after prolonged contact with a mild irritant (such as some soaps and detergents); the area may become raw if it is scratched.*

**D**ermatitis is often an allergic reaction of the skin, producing an acute local inflammation. This may be caused by contact with irritant substances, such as metals, perfumes, cosmetics or even plants, or it may be part of a general allergic or 'atopic' condition, often linked with asthma *(see p.52)* and hay fever *(see p.48)*. Dermatitis caused by direct contact can spread to distant parts of the body. Self-help and simple home remedies are a real must.

## 🌐 Call the doctor

*If the dermatitis is weeping and crusting, since it may be infected.*

### CONVENTIONAL MEDICINE

Moisturize your skin regularly. If the dermatitis is severe, consult a doctor, as treatment with steroid creams may be necessary.

DOSAGE: ADULTS AND CHILDREN Choose a non-perfumed moisturizer; apply as often as possible.

### NUTRITION

Many forms of dermatitis are triggered by foods: both by their natural constituents and by artificial food additives. Handling foods such as garlic, raw fish and mangoes is another common trigger. Avoiding all artificial additives is the first step towards healing. Then keep a food diary, noting when your skin looks better or worse. The most common irritant foods (in descending order) are milk and all dairy products, shellfish, eggs, citrus fruit, strawberries, red meat and wheat products.

A high intake of vitamins A and E, beta-carotene and essential fatty acids is very important, so drink a large glass of carrot juice every day. Eat plenty of broccoli, spinach, parsley, tomatoes, apricots, sunflower seeds and oil, oily fish, nuts, soya products, red and green peppers, oats, wheatgerm and brown rice. Drink copious amounts of water and eat parsley and celery to stimulate the kidneys.

## ❖ HOMEOPATHIC REMEDIES

🕭 **Kali arsenicosum 6c**
For itching that is intolerable. Worse for warmth, at night and for undressing. Skin dry and scaly.

🕭 **Kreosotum 6c**
For dermatitis on hands and backs of fingers, face and eyelids. Very itchy. Worse in evening. Better for warmth.

🕭 **Petroleum 6c**
For dry, leathery, rough skin with cracks. Burning and itching. Skin may be red, raw and bleed. Worse in winter.

**DOSAGE** 1 tablet daily. Maximum 2 weeks (see also Eczema on p.134).

## AROMATHERAPY

🕭 **Tea tree** (Melaleuca alternifolia)
🕭 **Lavender** (Lavandula angustifolia)
🕭 **Roman camomile** (Chamaemelum nobile)

Tea tree is antiviral, antifungal and antibacterial. Lavender and camomile are soothing, anti-inflammatory and painkilling.

**APPLICATION** Use in a bath and as a topical cream on the skin. Tea tree can also be used in the laundry of towels and facecloths (make sure the sufferer has separate items from the rest of the family), which will stop the spread of the infection. (See also Eczema on p.134 and Stress on p.36.)

## HERBAL REMEDIES

Borage and other herbs are useful in soothing the irritant rash of contact dermatitis.

**USE AND DOSAGE** Use a lotion made from equal amounts of borage juice and distilled witch hazel. Make fresh borage juice by pulping the leaves in a food processor, or it is available commercially.

Evening primrose or comfrey creams can also help; or apply the sap from a fresh Aloe vera leaf.

Internally, garlic has an antihistamine effect to combat the allergic response (use cloves in cooking or take up to 1g daily in capsules), while burdock and cleavers tea can be soothing.

### Prevention

*For contact dermatitis, avoid skin contact with nickel and metal alloys; perfumes, soaps, detergents and cosmetics are common causes, so buy hypoallergenic varieties. And avoid hair dyes, rubber gloves, many medicated creams and ointments and some plants, such as primulas, euphorbias and rue, if you are susceptible. Regular moisturizing of the skin is the most vital part of your daily routine.*

**BELOW** Aloe vera has many herbal uses and its sap may soothe dermatitis.

# Eczema

*Starts with a patch of itchy skin covered with small blisters, which may become red and raw if scratched; in long-standing eczema the skin may become thick, with accentuated markings; sometimes it causes flaky skin – as dandruff on the scalp.*

Those unfortunate people who suffer from asthma, hay fever and eczema are described as atopic. They may have to endure all these problems, and frequently pass them on to their children. There are many similarities between eczema and dermatitis *(see p.132)* and some conditions labelled dermatitis are in fact eczema.

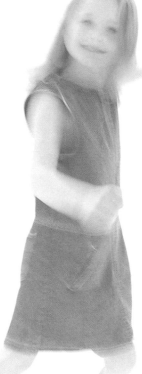

## CONVENTIONAL MEDICINE

Moisturize the skin regularly using bath oil, soap substitute or lotion. If eczema is severe, consult a doctor; you may need treatment with steroid creams.
DOSAGE: ADULTS AND CHILDREN Choose a non-perfumed moisturizer; apply as often as possible.

## HOMEOPATHIC REMEDIES

Consultation with a homeopath may be helpful.

### Arsenicum album 6c
For dry, rough, scaly skin. Itching and burning. Scratching until skin is raw briefly alleviates this.

### Graphites 6c
For rawness in bends of elbows and knees, and behind ears. Oozes pale fluid. Corners of mouth crack. Skin dry and hard.

### Sulphur 6c
For dry, burning, scaly skin. Scalp dry. Itching worse for scratching and water.
DOSAGE 1 tablet twice daily. Stop after 2 weeks or on improvement. Repeat if necessary.

## NUTRITION

Food is frequently a major factor in controlling the flare-up of symptoms, but is not a cure. In asthmatic children, one of the most common culprits is chemical additives – colourings, flavourings, preservatives and flavour enhancers – which should be avoided.

### Call the doctor
*If the eczema is weeping and crusting, as it may be infected.*

Early exposure to cow's milk is often the original cause of infantile eczema, so try to avoid giving cow's milk to babies for as long as possible.

All dairy products and citrus fruit can make eczema flare up, but the offending food is often very personal to the individual – from shellfish to strawberries, chocolate to cashew nuts. Compiling a food diary, and noting when the condition becomes better or worse, can supply pointers to the trigger foods; but unless these are few and not essential nutritionally, long-term exclusion diets should be undertaken only under professional guidance.

**ABOVE** Confectionery is often high in colourings, preservatives and other additives.

### HERBAL REMEDIES

Herbalists generally treat atopic eczema with cleansing herbal teas and limited use of creams.

USE AND DOSAGE Mix equal amounts of red clover, heartsease, burdock leaves, fumitory and stinging nettles, which will help to reduce inflammation, stimulate the digestion and circulation, and clear any toxins. Use 2tsp of the mixture to a cup of boiling water, three times a day.

Evening primrose used as an external cream or taken internally (2g per day) can also help.

Chickweed, marsh-mallow and camomile creams can all be beneficial.

> ### Caution
> Do not apply essential oils to broken, weeping skin without first getting professional advice.

### AROMATHERAPY

- Lavender *(Lavandula angustifolia)*
- Roman camomile *(Chamaemelum nobile)*
- Geranium *(Pelargonium graveolens)*
- Juniper *(Juniperus communis)*
- Rose *(Rosa damascena/Rosa centifolia)*
- Cedarwood *(Cedrus atlantica)*

All these oils are soothing and anti-inflammatory. Juniper is also detoxifying (it may make your condition worse before it gets better, but do persevere).

APPLICATION Mix calendula base oil or aqueous cream (available from chemists) with the oils, then rub them gently into the affected area. Alter the formula until you find one that helps your condition. Check for allergies *(see p.14)* and stress *(see p.36)*.

**BELOW** Keep a food diary to determine which foods – for instance, cow's milk – cause exzema to flare up.

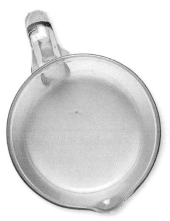

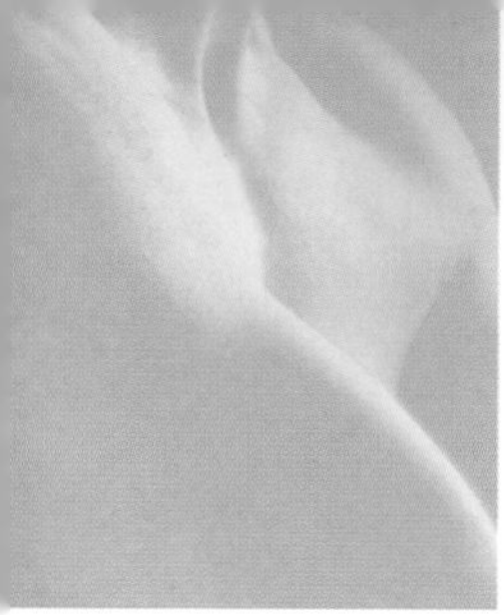

# Hives: urticaria

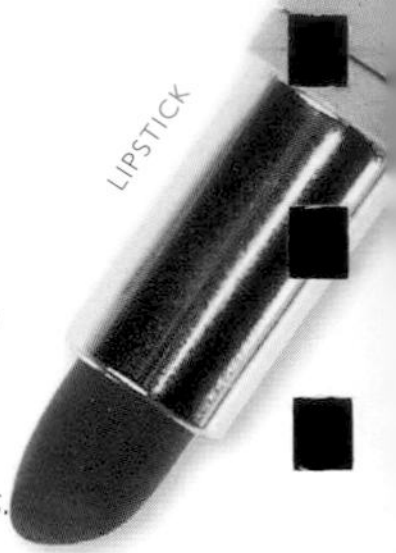

LIPSTICK

*An itchy rash that looks like nettle- or poison-ivy rash, affecting a small area of skin or even the whole body; tends to come and go, leaving no marks, and may improve after a few days or continue for months.*

**Hives – or urticaria, to give it its medical name – is also known as nettle-rash, as its appearance is similar to the lumpy skin eruptions caused by stinging nettles. It is an allergic reaction and can be caused by foods, contact with plants (not necessarily nettles), cosmetics, medications, any domestic cleaning chemicals, alcohol, sudden exposure to cold or hot air and, very often, by sunlight. Food additives and colourings are frequent culprits, but eruptions of these irritating lumps and bumps can also be triggered by stress and anxiety.**

**BELOW** Many foodstuffs are blamed for causing urticaria. Monitor your diet to see which affects you.

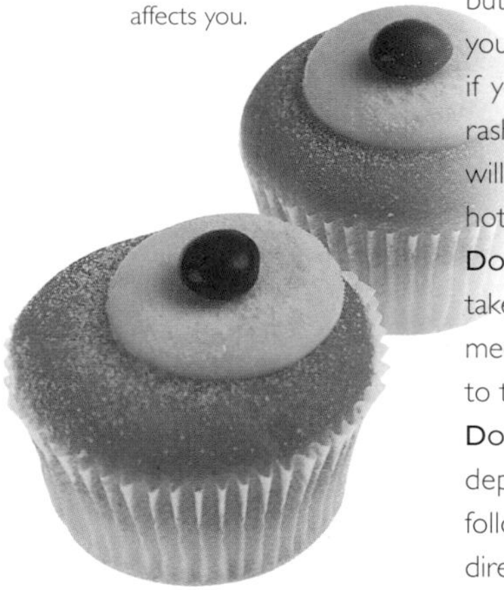

## CONVENTIONAL MEDICINE

If you know what triggers the rash, you can avoid it, but in most cases all you can do is try and reduce your symptoms. The rash will be more comfortable if you keep cool. Antihistamines may prevent the rash from developing, although some preparations will make you drowsy. Try calamine lotion to soothe hot, itchy skin.

**DOSAGE: ADULTS** Most antihistamine tablets are taken once a day; consult pack for details, or follow medical advice. Apply calamine lotion/cream directly to the skin as required.

**DOSAGE: CHILDREN** Doses of antihistamine syrup depend on the age of the child: consult pack, or follow medical advice. Apply calamine lotion/cream directly to the skin as required.

## NUTRITION

The only long-term treatment is to identify and then avoid the foods that cause attacks by following the exclusion diet *(see p.201)*. The most common irritating foods are shellfish, chocolate, strawberries, eggs, nuts, dairy products, wheat (rarely) and, very commonly, food additives (particularly tartrazine). Aspirin and its derivatives are another common

**Call the doctor**

*If the rash persists or if it becomes widespread over the body.*

factor in this condition. For those who have identi-fied aspirin as a culprit, it may be worth eliminating all foods that contain natural aspirin as well (most berries, dried and fresh fruit, some nuts and seeds). If your nettle-rash is triggered by sunlight, eat foods rich in beta-carotene: carrots, apricots, spinach, broccoli, peppers and tomatoes. Avoid Earl Grey tea (flavoured with bergamot) and buckwheat.

*STINGING NETTLE*

*DOCK LEAVES*

### AROMATHERAPY

- Roman camomile *(Chamaemelum nobile)*
- Lavender *(Lavandula angustifolia)*
- Melissa *(Melissa officinalis)*

Camomile and lavender soothe the irritation; melissa and camomile calm the allergic reaction.

**APPLICATION** Use in a light cream base to rub onto the irritated area; in a spray, if the area is too tender to be touched; or in water – either sponge the affected area down or use in the bath.

### HOMEOPATHIC REMEDIES

Severe allergic reactions require medical help.

- Urtica urens 30c

For nettle-rash, very itchy red blobs with a white centre. Allergic reactions, particularly to shellfish. Worse for cold bathing. Urticaria with joint pains. This is probably the most common remedy.

**DOSAGE** 1 tablet every 15 minutes until improved. Maximum ten doses.

**ABOVE** Dock leaves can help to soothe the pain of nettle-rash.

### HERBAL REMEDIES

Minor or occasional outbreaks can be soothed with camomile cream or borage juice, as well as with such traditional standbys as dock leaves, freshly sliced onion or crushed cabbage leaves.

**USE AND DOSAGE** For persistent problems, generally associated with food allergy, make a tea containing agrimony and camomile (2 parts each) with hearts-ease and stinging nettles (1 part each), to combat the action of histamine and improve resistance to allergens in the gut. Use 2tsp of the mixture per cup, three times daily.

**BELOW** Crabs and other shellfish are the most common irritating foods.

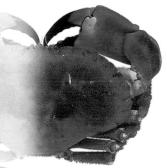

# Psoriasis

*Thick red patches of skin that are covered by silvery-white
scales, often starting on the knees and backs of the elbows,
or on the trunk of the body, but sometimes spreading to
cover most of the body surface.*

**P**soriasis is a chronic skin condition, which tends to run in families
and affects approximately one person in 50 in both Britain and the
United States, although it is much rarer in the black population. It
occurs because the skin cells are reproducing far more quickly than
normal – the normal cycle takes 311 hours, but in psoriasis it takes just
36. It is more common in smokers and heavy alcohol drinkers, although
it can start at any age, most frequently in the late twenties to thirties.
Attacks may start with a bacterial throat infection or follow a stressful
event; psoriasis can also be a reaction to some drugs.

**ABOVE** Use only non-perfumed moisturizers on affected skin.

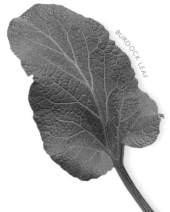

BURDOCK LEAF

### ✚ CONVENTIONAL MEDICINE

It is important to keep the skin well moisturized
using bath oil, soap substitute or lotion. Rehumidify
the air using a basin of water placed near radiators.
If the symptoms persist, seek medical advice – conventional treatment includes prescribed lotions,
shampoos and creams to put on the skin. In more
severe cases, treatment with ultraviolet light may
help those with psoriasis.

DOSAGE: ADULTS AND CHILDREN Choose a non-
perfumed moisturizer; apply as often as possible.

### HERBAL REMEDIES

Small areas of psoriasis often respond well to
cleavers cream.

USE AND DOSAGE Add 1 cup of strained cleavers
infusion to 1 cup of melted emulsifying ointment
(available from chemists) and stir constantly as it
cools and thickens.

Mix equal amounts of the roots of blue flag,
burdock and yellow dock for a decoction (1tsp
per cup) or use an infusion of cleavers, red clover
flowers and burdock leaf (2tsp per cup). Where stress
is a factor, add skullcap or passionflower to the mix.

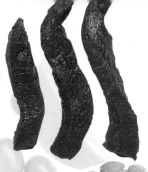

## AROMATHERAPY

- ⚜ Lavender *(Lavandula angustifolia)*
- ⚜ Basil *(Ocimum basilicum)*
- ⚜ Bergamot *(Citrus bergamia)*
- ⚜ Vetivert *(Vetiveria zizanoides)*

The body/mind connection is important: you have psoriasis, so you become stressed because it looks unsightly, and the stress only makes the psoriasis worse. Break the cycle with these de-stressing oils.
**APPLICATION** Good base oils are essential — refined avocado (or just ordinary avocado) or carrot oil. Add a few drops of essential oil to these if you do not want your aqueous cream base to be too greasy. Regular massage from a professional as well as localized self massage, will also help.

## HOMEOPATHIC REMEDIES

Consultation with a homeopath may be helpful.
- ⚜ Sepia 6c
For itchy psoriasis, not relieved by scratching. On elbows, backs of hands, palms. Scaly, but as soon as one scale comes off another forms.
- ⚜ Petroleum 6c
For dry, cracked, rough skin. Cracked ends of fingers. Worse in winter. Itching at night. Psoriasis on hands.
**DOSAGE** I tablet twice daily. Stop after 2 weeks or on improvement. Repeat if necessary.

**ABOVE** Orange and red fruit and pumpkin seeds are good for the skin, but some psoriasis sufferers find that fish and red meat worsen their condition.

## NUTRITION

Zinc, beta-carotene, vitamin D and omega-3 fatty acids are essential nutrients. Eat plenty of oily fish for its vitamin D and fatty acids; orange, red and dark green fruit and vegetables for beta-carotene; and shellfish, oysters and pumpkin seeds for zinc.

Although psoriasis is not an allergic condition, specific foods may aggravate it. Fish, shellfish, citrus fruit, red meat, dairy products, caffeine and alcohol are the most common triggers. If you notice any of these making your skin worse, try to avoid them. Avoid liver and other offal, because they can increase the body's production of complex chemicals, which (normally beneficial) may aggravate psoriasis.

### Prevention

*There is no specific way to prevent psoriasis, but it is often possible to keep it in check. Sunshine is known to be beneficial, and relaxation techniques may help, for stress is often a major factor. Supplements of vitamin D, beta carotene and zinc can also play a part.*

# Ringworm: tinea

*One or more round areas of scaly, slightly itchy, abnormal-looking skin; the centre of the abnormal area may look more normal, leading to the appearance of a ring; usually occurs on moist areas such as the armpits, groin and feet.*

**R**ingworm is an inflammatory infection of the skin caused by mould or fungi (and 90 per cent of all fungal infections are caused by the moulds *Microsporum epidermophyton* and *M. trichophyton*). Ringworm infections (so called because of the red patches with a raised outside edge, and nothing to do with worms), or tinea, thrive in areas of the body that are moist and warm. Home remedies work well in the treatment of this condition. Ringworm is a common complaint and highly contagious, as it is spread by direct physical contact. It can be acquired from horses, farmyard animals and cats *(Microsporum canis)*.

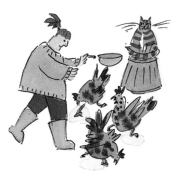

## CONVENTIONAL MEDICINE

Ringworm on the body can usually be treated effectively with antifungal creams. If the rash has not cleared up after two weeks, consult your doctor. Ringworm that affects the scalp or nails can be more difficult to treat and you should discuss it with your doctor.

DOSAGE: ADULTS AND CHILDREN Most creams are applied twice a day; consult pack for details.

## HOMEOPATHIC REMEDIES

∞ Tellurium 6c

For ringworm over whole body, lower limbs. May be more on left side. Itching worse after going to bed, for cool air and rest. Intersecting rings over whole body.

DOSAGE 1 tablet daily. Maximum 2 weeks.

## AROMATHERAPY

∞ Tea tree *(Melaleuca alternifolia)*
∞ Myrrh *(Commiphora molmol)*
∞ Lavender *(Lavandula angustifolia)*

Tea tree and myrrh are antifungal and will attack the fungus that causes ringworm. If lavender is the only oil you have, you can use this, as it has a slight fungicidal effect.

**APPLICATION** Apply as a compress; as a water spray (but not too near the eyes); or in a massage medium. Do be aware, however, that ringworm is infectious, and make sure that your hygiene is scrupulous, especially if you are applying oils to somebody else. Wash your hands well afterwards, using the oils in the hand wash.

THYME

### HERBAL REMEDIES

Tea tree, thyme and marigold all show antifungal activity and can be very effective for infections such as ringworm.

**USE AND DOSAGE** Apply tea-tree, thyme or marigold creams to affected areas three or four times a day.

If the scalp is affected, use a strained marigold infusion as a rinse, or add 5 drops of tea-tree or thyme oil to the rinsing water after shampooing (ideally combined with a strong soapwort infusion, which is very cleansing).

Internally, cleavers and chickweed tea will also help (1tsp of each per cup).

### NUTRITION

Poor nutrition, which results in a lowered natural resistance, can make anyone more susceptible to attack by these ubiquitous moulds and fungi. A diet rich in all the essential nutrients, especially vitamins A, C and E and the minerals zinc and selenium, is generally important for maintenance of the body's natural defences.

**BELOW** Raspberries are a rich and delicious source of vitamin C.

So eat plenty of orange and red fruit, dark green leafy vegetables and liver (but not if you are pregnant) for their vitamin A; citrus fruit and other fresh produce for their vitamin C; avocados, nuts, seeds and olive oil for their vitamin E; shellfish, oysters and pumpkin seeds for their zinc; and brazil nuts for their selenium. Regular consumption of garlic acts as a systemic fungicide and is a particularly important remedy if the ringworm has affected the finger- or toenails.

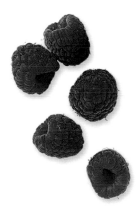

# Hair problems

*Flaking scalp — likely cause: dandruff; patches of complete hair loss — likely cause: Alopecia areata; generalized thinning and dry hair — likely cause: underactive thyroid gland; men's hair receding at temples — likely cause: male-pattern baldness.*

**H**air problems are frequently a sign of underlying illness, as hair is a true barometer of health. Many of the difficulties that arise are, however, simply the result of not caring for your hair properly. Most women lose hair after childbirth, but it does grow back again; the same is true – for men and women – after any serious illness.

## CONVENTIONAL MEDICINE

Excessive hair growth can be treated with bleaching, electrolysis or waxing, but can make dark hair look orange. Hair loss after pregnancy or due to *Alopecia areata* tends to regrow, although your doctor may get blood tests done, to ensure your thyroid gland is working normally. Male-pattern baldness can be treated, but the new hair is downy and falls out again if the treatment is stopped. Dandruff can be controlled with shampoo or lotion. In severe cases consult your doctor.

**DOSAGE: ADULTS AND CHILDREN** For male-pattern baldness, apply solution containing minoxidil twice a day. For dandruff, use a mild detergent shampoo once or twice a week. Products containing Ketoconazole are probably most effective. If using bleach, apply to hairy skin and leave, usually for 10–15 minutes; consult pack for details.

## HOMEOPATHIC REMEDIES

**Graphites 6c**

For crusts on scalp. Also eczema behind ears, which may be moist. Oozes sticky fluid.

**Oleander 6c**

For large white flakes falling from hair. Scalp dry or itchy. Psoriasis or cradle cap (in babies). Generally worse for eating oranges.

**DOSAGE** 1 tablet twice daily. Maximum 2 weeks.

## NUTRITION

Anaemia is one of the most frequent causes of hair loss, so eat plenty of iron-rich foods, like liver (not if you are pregnant), all other offal, wholegrain cereals, dark green leafy vegetables, eggs, dates and raisins. Vitamin C improves the absorption of iron, so eat fruit or vegetables at the same time. Vitamin E is also important for healthy hair growth, so eat avocados, nuts, seeds and olive oil on a regular basis. Reduce your intake of animal fat and sugar, as these can aggravate the production of sebum.

## HERBAL REMEDIES

**ABOVE** Cabbage contains iron, which is needed to prevent anaemia.

Herbs have a beneficial effect on a wide range of hair problems.

USE AND DOSAGE For dandruff, add 1–2 cups of rosemary or stinging-nettle infusion to the final rinse when shampooing.

Hair loss will sometimes respond to arnica, rosemary or southernwood (massage an infused oil into the scalp).

For dry hair, take marsh-mallow and burdock as a tea (1 tsp of each per cup).

For itchiness, use a final rinse of catmint or camomile infusion.

## AROMATHERAPY

- Rosemary *(Rosmarinus officinalis)*
- Roman camomile *(Chamaemelum nobile)*
- Lemon *(Citrus limon)*
- Grapefruit *(Citrus x paradisi)*
- Cedarwood *(Cedrus atlantica)*

Rosemary is usually used for dark hair and camomile for fair. Rosemary, lemon, grapefruit and cedarwood stimulate the circulation and balance the body's secretions, so reducing dandruff.

APPLICATION Add 2 drops of essential oil to the rinse water or a good vegetable oil, then massage into the scalp. Wrap your hair in clingfilm, then place a warm towel around it and leave for 2–3 hours or overnight. Then use a mild shampoo (not medicated), so that you do not damage the sebum balance.

> **Caution**
> Avoid rosemary oil if you have high blood pressure; if you have sensitive skin, keep lemon and grapefruit doses low as they may be irritant.

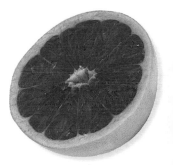

**BELOW** Add grapefruit oil to the final rinsing water when washing your hair to reduce dandruff.

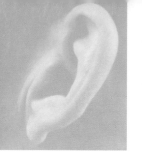

# Earache

*Throbbing pain and a fever, often during or after a cold; may be worse in an aeroplane; child may scream and pull at one ear – likely causes: middle-ear infection or catarrh; pain after syringing or swimming – likely cause: external ear infection.*

**E**arache is a common problem, especially in young children, and is generally caused by an infection. The Eustachian tube, which links the back of the nose and throat to the middle ear, can allow bacteria access to this sensitive region. The lining of the ear canal is very thin and easily damaged if you scratch or clean it overenthusiastically; an infected ear canal will be sore and often produces a discharge. Earache in children should always be regarded as serious and seen by your doctor, although it is not necessary to resort to antibiotics every time. Home remedies often avoid the need for stronger medication.

## 🌐 Call the doctor

*If earache persists in young children; if you have severe earache.*

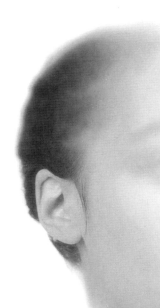

### ✚ CONVENTIONAL MEDICINE

To prevent damage to the ear canal, avoid cleaning the ears with cotton buds or scratching them too vigorously. A pain reliever will usually ease earache, but if the pain persists or if you have noticed any discharge from the ear, consult your doctor. In the meantime, keep the ear dry by putting cottonwool in it while showering.

**DOSAGE: ADULTS** 1–2 tablets of pain reliever at onset of pain, repeated every 4 hours; consult pack for details.

**DOSAGE: CHILDREN** Give regular doses of liquid pain reliever; consult pack, or follow medical advice.

### HERBAL REMEDIES

It is very important to avoid putting anything in the ear if there is the slightest risk that the eardrum has been perforated.

**USE AND DOSAGE** Warmed herbal oils (infused mullein or St John's wort, for instance) can be helpful as ear drops.

Alternatively, you can infuse a camomile teabag for a few minutes, then place it over the ear while it is still warm.

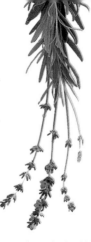

## ✿ HOMEOPATHIC REMEDIES

For recurrent earache, consult a qualified homeopath; if worsening, consult a doctor.

### ✍ Pulsatilla 6c

For heavy, pressing pain outwards from eardrum. Worse for applied heat. Thick, bland, smelly discharge. Child is miserable, clingy and wants cuddles.

### ✍ Chamomilla 6c

For severe, sharp pains in the ear driving person frantic. Child is irritable, angry, better for moving.

### ✍ Belladonna 6c

For sudden onset. Throbbing earache worse for heat. Hypersensitive hearing. Face very hot and red. Skin dry, may be delirious.

### ✍ Aconite 6c

For initial stages of earache. Pains may be worse in left ear.

DOSAGE 1 tablet every 4 hours for 2–3 days or until better.

**ABOVE** Lavender is a highly soothing oil and will help dull the pain of earache.

## ◌ AROMATHERAPY

### ✍ Lavender (Lavandula angustifolia)
### ✍ Roman camomile (Chamaemelum nobile)

Camomile is beneficial for a dull ache and lavender for sharp pain.

APPLICATION Put a drop of lavender on some cottonwool, then make a plug to place in the ear. Use camomile in a warm compress on the side of the face.

## ◌ NUTRITION

Children with recurrent earache may respond to a diet free of dairy products for a short period of time, as this seems to reduce the amount of mucus. But if your child is on a reduced dairy-product diet, seek professional advice to make sure there are no nutritional deficiencies.

Plenty of pineapple juice should be drunk for its healing enzymes, and citrus juices for their vitamin C. Otherwise, most children will want little food apart from light snacks, as swallowing often worsens the pain. For adults, decongestant spices such as cinnamon, ginger, chilli and mustard, will help.

> **Caution**
>
> Do not pour essential oil directly into the ear. If pus appears from the ear or you develop a fever, seek medical help. Always read pain-reliever packages carefully, and do not exceed the stated dose.

CINNAMON

MUSTARD

# Bad breath: halitosis

*An unpleasant smell on the breath; usually due to poor dental hygiene, but may also sometimes be caused by catarrh, constipation, the underproduction of saliva, smoking and drinking alcohol.*

Medically, bad breath is not usually very significant. Sometimes, however, it can be a pointer towards the diagnosis of more serious illness, such as liver failure, kidney disease or diabetes. Nearly always halitosis is the result of bad mouthkeeping – a build-up of plaque, infected gums, a tooth abscess, a rotting filling or lazy brushing. People often become obsessive about their breath, but dentists can now use electronic machines to measure the odours in exhaled breath. More people actually lose their teeth through gum disease than tooth decay *(see Gingivitis on p.150)*, so heed the following advice.

### ✚ CONVENTIONAL MEDICINE

Looking after teeth and gums by regular brushing, flossing and dental check-ups will help ensure that they are not responsible for unpleasant smells in the mouth. Sensible eating habits will often avoid the problem, but it is important to seek medical advice if there is no obvious cause.

### 🌿 HERBAL REMEDIES

Identifying the cause of bad breath is important.

USE AND DOSAGE If hyperacidity is to blame, then meadowsweet tea can help.

If sluggish digestion is at fault, then agrimony or fenugreek seeds (1tsp of herb to a cup of boiling water) can be useful.

Where bad breath is associated with catarrh, use either peppermint or tea-tree oil inhalants to sweeten the breath.

A traditional remedy is to chew a few lovage or fennel seeds.

An effective herbal mouth spray can be made by adding 5ml/1tsp each of tea-tree and rosemary oils to 100ml/3½fl oz of water and pouring into a spray bottle.

**ABOVE** Don't just mask bad breath; improve oral hygiene to eliminate it.

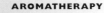

PEPPERMINT

### AROMATHERAPY

- Tea tree *(Melaleuca alternifolia)*
- Peppermint *(Mentha x piperita)*
- Thyme *(Thymus vulgaris)*
- Lemon *(Citrus limon)*
- Niaouli *(Melaleuca viridiflora)*

These oils kill off any unnecessary bacteria or viral infection that was in the mouth or throat, and which might be causing bad breath; they also freshen that area.

APPLICATION Use in a mouthwash or gargle.

> ### Caution
> Do not give mouthwashes containing essential oils to children.

### HOMEOPATHIC REMEDIES

Ensure that there is no serious cause for this particular complaint

- Pulsatilla 6c

For halitosis in the morning. Dry mouth with greasy taste. Not thirsty. Food may taste bitter.

- Kali bichromicum 6c

For offensive breath, sensation of a hair on the tongue. Thick saliva, ropy, yellow catarrh.

DOSAGE I tablet twice daily. Maximum 2 weeks.

### NUTRITION

Constipation is thought to be a common cause of bad breath and is easily remedied *(see p.96)*. Sinus infections, catarrh and chronic chest diseases can also be responsible *(see Catarrh on p.42, Sinusitis on p.50)*. Some people find the smell of garlic, onions, curries and other highly spiced food unpleasant, although all these foods are extremely healthy – so avoid them if you feel you must. Regular daily helpings of natural live yogurt, plenty of water and adequate amounts of fibre-containing foods – apples, pears, carrots, wholegrain cereals and beans – all improve the digestive function and will help bad breath. Eat plenty of broccoli, spinach and citrus fruits for their beta-carotene and vitamin C; ginger, horseradish, mustard and cinnamon for the sinuses; cut down on dairy products to reduce mucus. Chewing a few caraway seeds, mint leaves or a coffee bean may improve halitosis.

**BELOW** If bad breath is caused by poor digestion, boost the immune system by increasing your intake of high-fibre foods.

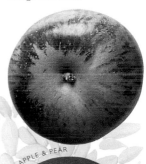
APPLE & PEAR

# Mouth ulcers

*Painful white craters, often with bright red borders, which may occur singly or in clusters and often recur; may appear on the tongue, the roof of the mouth, the groove between the gums and cheek, or elsewhere on the cheek.*

These are painful, irritating sore patches found inside the mouth, generally occurring on the inside of the lips (especially the lower one) and cheeks, although they can also appear on the gums and roof of the mouth. Their medical name is apthous ulcers and, though they are frequently caused by injury – biting the cheek or lip, badly fitting dentures or the jagged edge of a damaged tooth – there may equally be no clear cause. In rare cases they are associated with an underlying disorder affecting the whole digestive tract.

## 🌐 Call the dentist

*If you have an ulcer that recurs regularly in the same place, as it is quite likely to be caused by a dental problem; if an ulcer fails to heal after 3 weeks.*

### ✚ CONVENTIONAL MEDICINE

Most ulcers improve with no treatment after a few days, but may last for 2 weeks. Pastilles or ointment containing local anaesthetic can relieve the pain. These can be used with a paste containing steroid to hasten healing. Avoid hot, spicy or acidic foods.
DOSAGE: ADULTS AND CHILDREN Apply a paste containing steroid, combined with a local anaesthetic pastille or ointment, to the ulcer at regular intervals; consult pack for details. Salt-water mouthwashes used three or four times a day may be helpful.

### 💧 AROMATHERAPY

**Myrrh (Commiphora molmol)**
Myrrh helps to kill the pain and the infection, and stop it spreading. If you cannot get hold of myrrh essential oil, then myrrh tincture can be used instead of the myrrh and vodka solution.
APPLICATION Put 2 drops of myrrh in 5ml/1tsp of vodka, then dab directly onto the mouth ulcer.

### HERBAL REMEDIES

Suitable herbs for mouthwashes include sage, rosemary, marigold, raspberry leaves, cloves or camomile.
USE AND DOSAGE Myrrh and golden seal both taste

RASPBERRY LEAF

extremely bitter but can be very effective mouth-washes: buy the tinctures from a chemist or health-food store and add 10–20 drops of either to a glass of warm water.

Strengthen the immune system with regular garlic capsules to help recurrent ulcer problems.

## NUTRITION

As this condition is so often related to stress, it is important to have a diet that is extra-rich in all the B vitamins, so make sure that you eat plenty of meat, poultry, wheatgerm, brewer's yeast, leafy green vegetables, wholegrain cereals and whole-meal bread. Avoid foods that may be damaging to the delicate mucous membranes of the mouth, including very salty food, such as crisps, salted nuts, vinegar, pickles, chillies and very hot curries. If you have ulcers, all these foods will make them much more painful.

An effective natural remedy from southern Europe is to cut a clove of garlic in half, squeeze it until the oils appear, then dab on the mouth ulcer two or three times a day. Although this treatment stings and smells, the ulcer will normally disappear within 24 hours.

### Prevention

*Regular sufferers of mouth ulcers should take a daily dose of 5,000 IU of vitamin A, 200mg of vitamin E and 10mg of vitamin B.. It is also helpful to suck a combined vitamin C and zinc lozenge every day.*

## HOMEOPATHIC REMEDIES

Check with your doctor that there is no anaemia. Consult a homeopath to treat the tendency towards ulcers.

**Borax 6c**

For painful, white ulcers that bleed easily on con-tact, or when eating. Mouth hot and tender. Bitter taste in mouth.

**Nitric acid 6c**

For blisters and ulcers in mouth that bleed easily. Ulcers on tongue and soft palate. Tongue clean, red.

**Natrum muriaticum 6c**

For recurrent mouth ulcers, cold sores and colds. Person may be introverted and easily hurt.

**DOSAGE** I tablet twice daily until improved. Maximum 5 days.

**BELOW** Spicy and salty food can irritate mouth ulcers, so try to avoid it.

# Gingivitis

*Characterized by sore gums, which may be red and bleed
easily when you clean your teeth; associated with tartar and
plaque around the margin of the gum; needs treating to
prevent eventual loss of teeth.*

ar more teeth are lost through gum disease than through tooth
decay, and gingivitis – the condition when the gums bleed very
easily, and dental plaque and tartar accumulate around the gum margin – is by far the most common cause of gum disease. If gingivitis is left
untreated, then pockets of infected pus can develop at the base of
teeth, followed eventually by abscesses and loose teeth, which may
eventually fall out. Good oral hygiene is essential to the prevention of
this painful condition, but home remedies can make an extremely
effective cure once infection occurs.

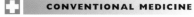

## CONVENTIONAL MEDICINE

Antiseptic mouthwashes and pain relievers may
help in the first instance. Seek the advice of a dentist or hygienist if the symptoms persist.

**DOSAGE: ADULTS** 1–2 tablets of pain relievers at
onset of pain, repeated every 4 hours; consult pack.
Use a recommended mouthwash twice a day.

**DOSAGE: CHILDREN** Give regular doses of liquid pain
reliever; consult pack, or follow medical advice. Use
a recommended mouthwash twice a day.

## AROMATHERAPY

- Myrrh *(Commiphora molmol)*
- Tea tree *(Melaleuca alternifolia)*
- Thyme *(Thymus vulgaris)*
- Fennel *(Foeniculum vulgare)*

These oils are all healing and help to stop infection;
thyme is antiseptic and myrrh is antimicrobial; tea
tree helps build up the body's immune system.

**APPLICATION** Use in a mouthwash, putting a few
drops of essential oil into a cup of warm water.
Alternatively, massage myrrh tincture into the gums
to improve the circulation (make sure your hands
are very clean before you do this).

## NUTRITION

It is the fibrous, as well as the nutritional, content of your food that is important in treating gingivitis. The massaging effect of biting on apples, pears, celery and raw carrots stimulates the blood flow to the margins of the gums and prevents the development of plaque, which is a haven for bacteria. Unfortunately, when this condition develops, the gums bleed easily, making the consumption of raw foods quite painful, and so a vicious circle starts.

Eat plentiful daily amounts of citrus fruit and all other fresh produce for their vitamin C. Eat as little sugar as possible and try to clean your teeth immediately after eating any high-sugar foods. If this is not possible, then chewing sugar-free gum for 15 minutes will help. And 1tsp of salt added to a glass of hot water makes a cheap, effective mouthwash.

APPLES

## HOMEOPATHIC REMEDIES

**Mercurius solubilis 6c**
For inflamed, bleeding gums. Produces lots of saliva. Breath is offensive and teeth may be loose. Metallic taste in mouth. Mouth moist but person is thirsty.

**Phosphorus 6c**
For gums that bleed easily and ulcerate. Bleeding after tooth extraction.

**Nitric acid 6c**
For teeth that become loose; spongy, bleeding gums. Tongue clean, red. May have ulcers on palate.
**DOSAGE** 1 tablet three times daily. Maximum 1 week.

### Caution
Some mouthwashes may cause brown stains on the teeth, which will improve when the mouthwash is stopped.

**BELOW** Supplement your oral-hygiene routine with a herbal mouthwash.

## HERBAL REMEDIES

Herbal mouthwashes can help to tonify and improve gum tissues, as well as combating infection and soothing ulceration.
**USE AND DOSAGE** Use a cooled, well-strained infusion or decoction containing herbs like echinacea, lady's mantle, marigold, marjoram, rosemary, sage or tormentil (2tsp per cup).

Take echinacea or golden seal capsules in order to boost the immune system.

MARJORAM

# Toothache

*Pain around a tooth; short bursts of pain, with inflammation of tooth pulp – likely cause: caries; long periods of pain, or sudden, severe pain – likely cause: inflamed pulp; intense, throbbing pain with sensitive gum – likely cause: abscess.*

Toothache is usually the result of poor mouthkeeping. Scrupulous attention to oral hygiene – proper flossing, careful brushing and a reduced consumption of canned fizzy drinks and sugar in general – represents the first step. Next come regular visits to your dentist. But many of the problems associated with toothache can be avoided by healthy eating. Dental caries (tooth decay), an abscess or gingivitis *(see p.150)* may be the cause of the pain. See your dentist! Weeks of painkillers will keep you going until the tooth pulp dies off and the pain stops, but then you will almost certainly lose the tooth.

## Caution

*Always read pain-reliever packages carefully, and do not exceed the stated dose.*

### CONVENTIONAL MEDICINE

Take a pain reliever as necessary to ease the toothache, and contact your dentist.

**DOSAGE: ADULTS** 1–2 tablets of pain relievers at onset, repeated every 4 hours; consult pack.

**DOSAGE: CHILDREN** Give regular doses of liquid pain reliever; consult pack, or follow medical advice.

### HOMEOPATHIC REMEDIES

This condition requires dental assessment.

**Chamomilla 30c**
Teething remedy for children. Person is intensely irritable, has intolerable pains and cries angrily. Child has to be carried constantly. Better for warm food.

**Coffea 30c**
For toothache eased with ice-cold water.

**Plantago 30c**
For teeth that are sore to touch, swelling in cheeks. Produces a lot of saliva. Worse for cold air and contact. Better for eating.

**Magnesium carbonicum 30c**
For toothache in pregnancy. Teeth very sensitive to touch. Worse at night. Pain from cutting wisdom teeth.

**DOSAGE** 1 tablet hourly for six doses, as needed.

## NUTRITION

Dental problems can be avoided by healthy eating, although this must be combined with good oral hygiene. Eat plentiful daily amounts of citrus fruit and all other fresh produce, as vitamin C is the most important single nutrient; crisp foods like apples, raw carrots and celery, which massage the gums when you chew; olive oil, sunflower-seed oil and sprouted seeds for their vitamin A; carrots, dark green leafy vegetables and liver (not if you are pregnant) for their vitamin A. Ensure that you reduce your intake of sugar, which is your gums' worst enemy – eat as little as possible and try to clean your teeth immediately after you have had any high-sugar foods.

## HERBAL REMEDIES

For abscesses and similar infections, strong antibiotic herbs – especially Chinese figwort (Xuan Shen), forsythia berries and echinacea – can sometimes solve the problem completely.

USE AND DOSAGE These antibiotic herbs are best taken in tinctures (5ml/1tsp three times daily).

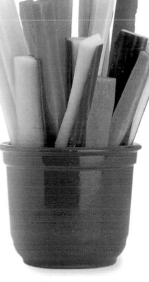

ABOVE Crunchy vegetables such as celery can help to improve the condition of your gums.

## AROMATHERAPY

◦ Clove (Syzygium aromaticum)
◦ Roman camomile (Chamaemelum nobile)
These oils only represent first-aid help until dental treatment can be organized. Clove has an anaesthetic effect and is also a strong antiseptic. Camomile is soothing and helps to kill the pain.

APPLICATION Dip a piece of cottonwool into some clove oil, roll it into a ball and stick it into the painful part of the tooth. You can also rub clove oil around the gum, or even hold a clove in the mouth. If you have mild toothache, then a warm camomile compress on the facial area is very soothing.

### Prevention

*Good oral hygiene, low consumption of sugars and high-sugar foods and healthy eating are all you need to prevent tooth problems leading to toothache.*

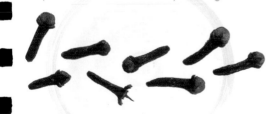

LEFT Cloves can provide a drug-free alternative treatment for toothache.

# Conjunctivitis

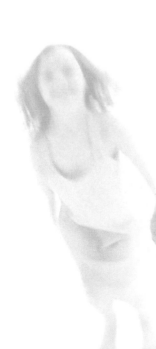

*Typical symptoms are eyes that have a red or puffy appearance, and a gritty feeling; a watery or sticky discharge; eyes that are often itchy; symptoms may affect either one or both eyes.*

**T**his acute inflammatory condition of the mucous membrane that covers the white of the eye and the inner surface of the eyelids, which is known as the conjunctiva, is caused by an infection or allergy. A foreign body in the eye can also result in the appearance of similar symptoms. Conjunctivitis can be serious and is extremely infectious, particularly in close-knit communities.

## CONVENTIONAL MEDICINE

For minor infections, bathe the eyes with water that has been boiled and then cooled. If this does not help, then antibiotic drops or ointment may be helpful. For allergic conjunctivitis, anti-histamine eye-drops can ease the symptoms.

**DOSAGE: ADULTS AND CHILDREN** Pull down the lower lid and insert antibiotics or ointment; consult pack for details, or follow medical advice. Continue the treatment for 48 hours after the symptoms have resolved themselves.

## HOMEOPATHIC REMEDIES

If the following remedies produce no improvement, seek medical help.

**Apis 6c**
For swollen, red, puffy eyelids. White of eye red, hot tears, intolerance of light.

**Argentum nitricum 6c**
For yellow or white discharge, white of eye red. Babies with sticky eye.

**Pulsatilla 6c**
For white or yellow discharge. Lids inflamed. Itching and burning. Person may be weepy and feel sorry for themselves.

**Euphrasia 6c**
For white of eye that is red, constantly watering. Tears burn, lids swollen.

**DOSAGE** I tablet every 4 hours. Maximum 2 days. Euphrasia tincture can be diluted (2 drops in an eggcup of cooled boiled water) to make a solution with which to bathe the eye.

### HERBAL REMEDIES

Herbal eyebaths are soothing and easy to make. Suitable herbs are marigold flowers, eyebright, camomile flowers, rose petals, raspberry leaves, elderflowers and fumitory.

**USE AND DOSAGE** Add 1tsp of herb to a cup of boiling water, then simmer gently to sterilize for 5 minutes before straining well. Allow to cool and then use the solution in an eyebath.

Take echinacea (6 x 200mg capsules every day) to combat any infection and strengthen the immune system.

**ABOVE** Carrots are rich in vitamin A, while cucumber can relieve inflammation caused by conjunctivitis.

### AROMATHERAPY

No essential oils can be used in the vicinity of the eyes.

### NUTRITION

Foods that are rich in beta-carotene, which the body converts to vitamin A, are important for all eye conditions — so eat orange and red fruit, all dark green leafy vegetables, carrots and liver (but not if you are pregnant). Thin slices of cucumber or used, cold teabags placed over the closed eyes for 6 minutes will help to relieve the inflammation caused by conjunctivitis.

**Prevention**

*Take care to protect your eyes by wearing suitable goggles when you are doing DIY tasks at home that might give rise to a foreign body getting into the eye.*

ECHINACEA

**LEFT** If home remedies such as echinacea and eyebright do not provide any relief, then consult a doctor without delay.

EYEBRIGHT

# Styes

*Starts with a painful lump near an eyelash; the pain may become severe and throbbing and the stye may discharge pus.*

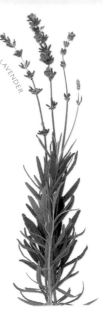

LAVENDER

**A** stye is an abscess in the tiny gland that is located at the bottom of each eyelash. It comes to a head or 'point' on the outside of the lid and can cause extreme inflammation of the eyelids. Infection may spread to the eye itself, so styes are not to be treated lightly. They tend to be more common in those who have low resistance and those in poor general health.

### CONVENTIONAL MEDICINE

A stye will often get better with no treatment except pain relievers. If it does not, then a course of antibiotics may be necessary.

**DOSAGE: ADULTS** 1–2 tablets of pain relievers at onset, repeated every 4 hours.

**DOSAGE: CHILDREN** Give regular doses of liquid pain reliever; consult pack or follow medical advice.

### HERBAL REMEDIES

Marigold or eyebright decoctions can be used to bathe the affected area, or a little marigold cream will help.

**USE AND DOSAGE** Simmer the decoction for 5 minutes to ensure a sterile mixture for bathing the eye.

If styes are recurrent and linked to overwork, take Siberian ginseng in the build-up to any especially stressful period.

### HOMEOPATHIC REMEDIES

**Staphysagria 6c**

For recurrent styes, and styes that leave a hard, inflamed area in the skin.

**DOSAGE** 1 tablet every 4 hours until stye is improved. Maximum 4 days.

# Childhood Illnesses

Children are naturally resilient, but all of them at one time or another will fall prey to illnesses like tonsillitis, measles or whooping cough, and there is nothing more miserable than seeing a child in discomfort and feeling that there is little you can do to help. However, although conventional medicine (and particularly vaccination) has an important role to play, there is much else that you can do at home to help alleviate the condition; and, even before illness takes hold, you can raise a child's resistance to infection and boost his or her natural immunity.

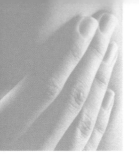

# Tonsillitis

*A sore throat, accompanied by difficulty in swallowing; swollen glands in the neck; a coated tongue; fever; the tonsils themselves may be red and inflamed, and covered in yellow spots of pus.*

Tonsillitis is an acute infection of the tonsils, usually caused by a virus, although it may be bacterial. When the tonsils become infected they look red and angry, but they are simply doing their job – trapping invading organisms before you inhale them. Tonsillitis occurs mostly in children, especially when first exposed to a range of bugs on starting school. Sometimes the problem becomes chronic, and it may also affect adults. Severe infections may need treatment with anti-biotics (which are only effective against bacterial infections), but home remedies are a powerful aid to reducing pain and speedier healing.

**BELOW** Children might need antibiotics to ward off severe tonsillitis.

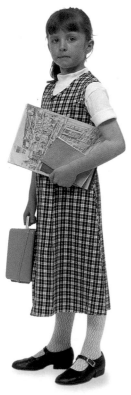

### ✚ CONVENTIONAL MEDICINE

Most infections will improve without any treatment, but doctors prescribe antibiotics for bacterial infections if symptoms have been present for sev-eral days. Painkillers can relieve the sore throat and fever, and can be dissolved to produce an anaes-thetic gargle. Lozenges and hot drinks can be soothing. Recurrent infections may be prevented by surgery to remove the tonsils.

**DOSAGE: ADULTS** Antibiotic tablets up to four times a day; follow medical advice; complete the course.

**DOSAGE: CHILDREN** Give antibiotic syrup up to four times a day. Dose depends on age and weight of child; follow medical advice; complete the course.

### 🍎 NUTRITION

During a bout of tonsillitis swallowing can be excru-ciatingly painful, so give liquidized vegetable soups made with carrots, sweet potatoes and broccoli for their beta-carotene; shredded cabbage and toma-toes for their vitamin C; and leeks, onions and garlic for their antiseptic qualities. Try crushing 2 peeled cloves of garlic into a jar of runny honey – a tea-spoonful can be given every couple of hours.

Drink plenty of hot water, honey and lemon, together with unsweetened fruit juices. Home-made ice lollies of pure frozen pineapple juice are easy to suck, and the bromelain in the pineapple helps reduce both the swollen glands and tonsils.

## HERBAL REMEDIES

Mild cases will generally respond well to gargling with sage and echinacea tinctures (5ml/1tsp of each) diluted in a glass of warmed pineapple juice. Other suitable gargles are raspberry-leaf tea, marsh cudweed infusion, or 10 drops of thuja or golden seal tinctures in a glass of water.

USE AND DOSAGE Support the immune system with echinacea capsules (up to 600mg four times a day).

Drink a mixture of camomile, cleavers and sage tea (equal amounts, 2tsp of the mixture per cup) to help the lymphatic system.

## HOMEOPATHIC REMEDIES

Recurrent problems are best treated by a homeopath.

☙ **Phytolacca 30c**
For dark red or purple tonsils with grey or white pus. Pain goes to ear on swallowing. Worse on right side, worse for warm drinks. Better for cold drinks.

☙ **Lachesis 30c**
For purple tonsils. Wakes with sore throat or worse after sleep. Worse on left side, for swallowing liquids and saliva. May start on left side and move to right.

DOSAGE 1 tablet every 2 hours for three doses, then every 4 hours. Maximum 2 days.

## AROMATHERAPY

☙ **Thyme** *(Thymus vulgaris)*
☙ **Lavender** *(Lavandula angustifolia)*
☙ **Tea tree** *(Melaleuca alternifolia)*
Tea tree and thyme both fight the infection; lavender and thyme have a slightly anaesthetic effect.

APPLICATION Use in steam inhalations or in a warm compress on the throat area. If other symptoms occur, such as earache, headache or abdominal pain, then look under the appropriate ailment.

**Call the doctor**
*If you are unable to swallow saliva.*

**BELOW** Try camomile teas as a healing drink, or for gargling.

# Measles

*Characterized by a fever; runny nose; red, watery eyes; cough;*
*and swollen glands. After 3–4 days an itchy rash develops,*
*starting at the head and spreading downwards, fading*
*after 3 days.*

This highly contagious viral infection causes a rash and attacks the respiratory system. The concerted effort to vaccinate all school children now makes it a much rarer complaint than it used to be, but it is still a very serious illness and should not be taken lightly. Home remedies are not a substitute for your doctor's advice, but they can make a child much more comfortable. Children with measles must be isolated; the infectious period lasts from the first symptoms – catarrh, conjunctivitis, high fever and complete misery – until 5 days after the first appearance of the rash. It can take up to 3 weeks to develop symptoms after being in contact with someone with measles.

## CONVENTIONAL MEDICINE

Treat the fever with pain relievers, and use calamine lotion to help soothe itchy skin.

DOSAGE: ADULTS 1–2 tablets of pain relievers at onset of fever, repeated every 4 hours; consult pack for details. Apply calamine lotion/cream directly to the skin as required.

DOSAGE: CHILDREN Give regular doses of liquid pain reliever; consult pack for details, or follow medical advice. Apply calamine lotion/cream directly to the skin as required.

## HERBAL REMEDIES

Herbs can ease symptoms and combat the infection, to support orthodox treatments.

USE AND DOSAGE Make an infusion of equal amounts of hyssop, marsh-mallow, catmint and ribwort plantain (½–1tsp of the mix per cup, depending on the age of the child) and sweeten with a little honey, to soothe coughs and lubricate dry throats.

Use well-strained, cooled infusions of eyebright or self-heal to bathe sore eyes, or to soak a cloth for use as a compress.

Use lemon-balm tea to help reduce fevers.

## NUTRITION

Few children with measles will feel like eating in the early stages, but as soon as they do, foods rich in vitamins A and C should be given as light meals. Puréed carrot with a poached egg; sweet potatoes cut into chips and roasted; dried apricots puréed with yogurt and stirred into a packet of jelly before setting; kiwi fruit with their tops sliced off and eaten like a boiled egg…these foods are easy to eat and will boost the immune system and protect the eyes.

Fruit juices – especially pineapple and orange – should be given in large amounts, diluted 50:50 with water. And leeks, garlic and onions are all protective against the secondary chest infection that often accompanies measles.

## HOMEOPATHIC REMEDIES

If the condition worsens, consult a doctor.

### Morbillinum 30c
After contact with measles, this remedy may help to prevent the disease. Take every 8 hours.

### Bryonia 6c
For dryness, hotness. Cough with headache. Worse for any motion. May be used before rash appears.

### Pulsatilla 6c
For miserable, clingy child, who wants to be cuddled. Bland, creamy discharge from eyes. Not thirsty. Temperature not very high.

DOSAGE 1 tablet every 4 hours until improved. Maximum 5 days.

## AROMATHERAPY

### Tea tree (Melaleuca alternifolia)
### Eucalyptus (Eucalyptus radiata)
### Roman camomile (Chamaemelum nobile)
### Lavender (Lavandula angustifolia)

These oils help to fight infection and are soothing.

APPLICATION Vaporize the sickroom to stop the virus being spread by airborne germs. Use the oils with a little warm water to sponge down the patient, or to spray into the air. Also use them as inhalations, especially if there is a sore throat.

ABOVE Tempt convalescing children with foods that are easy – and fun – to eat.

### Caution
Watch out for fits caused by very high temperatures and the possibility of meningitis, eye problems and secondary infections. Read pain-reliever packages carefully, and do not exceed the stated dose. Take Morbillinum for three doses only.

# German measles: rubella

*Mild fever; sore throat; and swollen glands, particularly behind the ears; the rash lasts 2–3 days, usually starting on the face and spreading downwards; individual spots may join together to produce a more generally flushed skin.*

The only significant thing about this mild, infectious disease is the risk it carries in pregnancy. Today most children are vaccinated against rubella (the medical term), but any child who does catch German measles must be kept away from all pregnant women, because of the risk to the unborn foetus – including deafness, blindness, heart and lung defects, and even death. Many women in the earliest stages of pregnancy may be unaware they are pregnant. Children with the illness must be kept at home during the infectious period, which lasts from the start of symptoms until at least 1 week after the rash appears.

## Call the doctor

*If German measles is suspected, since it is a notifiable disease; if you are pregnant, have been in contact with rubella and are not sure of your immune status.*

### CONVENTIONAL MEDICINE

If you have this common viral infection, you should rest if you feel unwell and avoid contact with other people, particularly school-age children and pregnant women. Although most women have had rubella or been immunized, if you are pregnant and worried that you have the illness, or have been in contact with someone with rubella, you should contact your doctor.

### HERBAL REMEDIES

Plenty of fluids are needed and herbal teas are ideal: they can be sweetened or flavoured with honey (use pasteurized for very young children), lemon, licorice or a little peppermint essence. Many soothing, cooling herbs are suitable, including lemon balm, camomile, catmint, marigold, sage and hyssop.
USE AND DOSAGE Elderflowers, marigold and camomile make a good combination; use ½–2tsp per cup of water (depending on age).

Echinacea capsules (100–600mg daily) will help combat the infection of German measles.

Sage, agrimony, cleavers or cinnamon tea helps to ease sore throats and swollen glands.

## AROMATHERAPY

- Lavender *(Lavandula angustifolia)*
- Roman camomile *(Chamaemelum nobile)*
- Tea tree *(Melaleuca alternifolia)*
- Eucalyptus *(Eucalyptus radiata)*

Camomile and lavender help to ease any irritation from the rash. Tea tree and eucalyptus, when burnt or vaporized, help to prevent the virus from spreading.

**APPLICATION** Use camomile and lavender in the bath. They can also be used (as can tea tree) in warm water to sponge children down, if they are getting clammy and distressed. Burn or vaporize the eucalyptus and the tea tree; alternatively use them in a water spray.

**ABOVE** Camomile can be used to ease an irritating rash or it may be added to bath water.

## HOMEOPATHIC REMEDIES

This is usually a mild disease and does not require treatment. If a woman has not been immunized to German measles and may have been exposed to it, then Rubella 30c, taken every 12 hours for three doses only, may help.

## NUTRITION

Fluids are absolutely vital. Drink plenty of diluted fresh citrus juices for their immune-boosting vitamin C, pineapple juice for its soothing enzymes (cartons of pineapple juice are fine); and herbal teas – camomile, lime blossom and elderflower (sweetened with honey if desired) are all ideal.

### Caution

*If German measles is contracted during the first 3 months of pregnancy, then the effects on the developing foetus can be catastrophic. Read pain-reliever packages carefully, and do not exceed the stated dose.*

### Prevention

*There is no way to prevent German measles, apart from vaccination. But it is important, as always, to maintain your child's general immunity in as strong a state as possible.*

**ABOVE** Sage tea makes a soothing remedy for rubella.

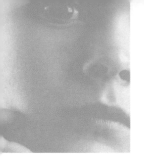

# Mumps

*Tiredness; mild fever; sore throat and pain on swallowing; swollen glands under the jaw; tender testicles in boys; a painful swelling in front of and below the ears after a couple of days – the temperature rises rapidly.*

This highly contagious viral infection mostly affects children between the ages of 4 and 14. It starts with general malaise and fever, followed by a painful swelling of the salivary gland on one side of the face. In 70 per cent of sufferers it goes on to affect the gland on the other side of the face, too. The incubation period lasts 14–21 days and sufferers are infectious (via coughs and sneezes or saliva) for 7 days before, and until 9 days after, the first swelling appears. The main complication is a condition called orchitis – swelling of the testicles – which occurs in 25 per cent of boys who catch the disease.

## CONVENTIONAL MEDICINE

Use a simple pain reliever to reduce the fever and ease the symptoms. Eat soft food and drink plenty of liquids.

**DOSAGE: ADULTS** 1–2 tablets of pain relievers at onset of fever, repeated every 4 hours; consult pack.

**DOSAGE: CHILDREN** Give regular doses of liquid pain reliever; consult pack for details, or follow medical advice.

**BELOW** Particular care must be given to boys who contract mumps.

## HERBAL REMEDIES

Swollen glands may be eased by a mixture of cleavers, thyme and marigold.

**USE AND DOSAGE** Mix equal amounts of the herbs and make an infusion (½–2tsp per cup, depending on the child's age); sweeten to taste with honey and a tiny pinch of chilli powder or cayenne. Repeat every 2 hours.

Take echinacea to combat the infection; if the testicles are affected use agnus-castus (10 drops of tincture in water three times daily).

Lemon balm or St John's wort infusion can be used externally in compresses applied to the face and throat, and to bathe swollen glands.

## NUTRITION

Getting sufficient calories into the child is the main difficulty, and soft or liquidized foods and drinks are best. Give plenty of vegetable juices diluted with warm water, apple or pear juice, purées of carrot and potato, liquidized yogurt with honey, fresh non-citrus fruit like dried apricots, mangoes and pawpaws which are both nutritious and healing. Pineapple juice – rich in the enzyme bromelain, which is anti-inflammatory and has a high content of natural sugars – will help, too. As soon as possible, give scrambled eggs; rice or tapioca puddings; pasta; mashed potato or avocado; real ice cream; minced chicken; and lots of bananas. A soluble vitamin C tablet (500mg) should be given every day. Avoid acidic fruit juices, as these increase the flow of saliva, which is very painful.

## HOMEOPATHIC REMEDIES

✎ Pulsatilla 6c

For use if the illness lingers; if there are complications of breasts swelling in girls or testicles swelling in boys (in which case, consult a doctor).

✎ Lachesis 6c

For swollen left side of face, which is sensitive to touch. Person tries to move away if someone tries to touch it. Sore throat, cannot swallow.

DOSAGE I tablet every 2 hours for six doses, then four times daily. Maximum 3 days.

## AROMATHERAPY

✎ Lavender (Lavandula angustifolia)
✎ Roman camomile (Chamaemelum nobile)
✎ Tea tree (Melaleuca alternifolia)
✎ Niaouli (Melaleuca viridiflora)
✎ Lemon (Citrus limon)

Lavender and camomile are soothing and help to kill the pain. The other oils help to combat infection.

APPLICATION Put into an oil or a lotion to smooth gently over the affected area, or use as a compress for swollen areas. Air sprays or vaporization will help stop the spread of airborne germs.

**ABOVE** Liquidized fruit is a palatable way to tempt youngsters to eat.

**Caution**

*Orchitis generally affects just one testicle, with few complications, but if both testicles are severely affected there is considerable risk of sterility – seriously increased if it occurs in adults. Always read pain-reliever packages carefully, and do not exceed the stated dose.*

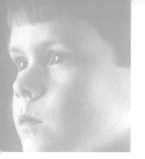

# Chickenpox

*Typified by a low fever, vomiting and general aches in some cases; small raised spots, breaking out first on the trunk, then on the face and limbs; crops of itchy blisters then affect the skin, eyes and mouth – they gradually crust and form scabs.*

his highly infectious illness is caused by the *Herpes zoster* virus and is most common in children. If they have been in contact with someone who is infected, it may be 2–3 weeks before symptoms appear. Although uncomfortable and irritating – the most serious side-effect is usually the scars left after picking the spots – some children may be quite poorly if they have a severe infection. In adults, however, chickenpox can be extremely serious and debilitating and may lead to acute pneumonia. Those who contract chickenpox must avoid scratching, to prevent the spread of infection and the risk of scars.

## CONVENTIONAL MEDICINE

Treat the fever with pain relievers, and use calamine lotion to soothe itchy skin. More severe infections can be treated with antiviral drugs, which may also be used in the early stages for adults.

**DOSAGE: ADULTS** 1–2 tablets of pain relievers at the onset of fever, repeated every 4 hours; consult pack for details. Apply calamine lotion/cream directly to the skin.

**DOSAGE: CHILDREN** Give regular doses of liquid pain reliever; consult pack for details, or follow medical advice. Apply calamine lotion/cream directly to the skin as required.

## HOMEOPATHIC REMEDIES

**Rhus toxicodendron 6c**
For intense itching, better for warm applications. Small watery blisters. This is the first remedy to try.

**Antimonium tartaricum 6c**
For spots that are slow to come out. Person is drowsy, sweaty. May have a cough with a rattly chest, but does not bring up any actual mucus.

**Antimonium crudum 6c**
For chickenpox and upset stomach. Person is

irritable, sulky. Cries when touched, looked at or washed. Tongue has a white coat.

**DOSAGE** 1 tablet every 2–4 hours until condition improves. Maximum 5 days.

### HERBAL REMEDIES

Herbs can ease the fever associated with chickenpox and soothe its rash.

**USE AND DOSAGE** To ease fevers and irritability, use a tea made from equal parts of boneset, elderflower and camomile (½–2tsp per cup, depending on patient's age, three times a day).

Rashes can be soothed with a wash made by mixing borage juice (30ml/2tbsp) with standard chickweed infusion (100ml/3½fl oz) and distilled witch hazel (25ml/1fl oz). Apply gently with a cotton wool swab as required.

Taking up to 6 × 200mg echinacea capsules daily will help combat the infection.

ELDERFLOWER

### NUTRITION

Take plenty of fluids, especially pineapple juice – which is rich in the enzyme bromelain – diluted with water (50:50), camomile tea and water itself. A short fast (24–48 hours) will boost the body's white-cell count and help to fight the infection.

### AROMATHERAPY

- Lavender *(Lavandula angustifolia)*
- Roman camomile *(Chamaemelum nobile)*
- Eucalyptus *(Eucalyptus radiata)*
- Bergamot *(Citrus bergamia)*

Bathing in these oils or rubbing in a lotion containing them will relieve itching. Vaporization will help stop the spread of the virus, so that hopefully other people will not catch it.

**APPLICATION** Use in lukewarm baths, vaporizers and sprays. Immerse the child in a lukewarm bath containing 1 drop of any of the above oils (but not all) every 2 hours. Regular bathing is also soothing for adults with chickenpox, who may be quite ill.

### Caution

*Always read pain-reliever packages carefully, and do not exceed the stated dose.*

**BELOW** Herbal teas can soothe itching and bring down fever.

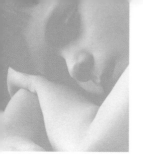

# Whooping cough

*Sneezing; watery red eyes; sore throat; mild fever; cough, with irregular bouts of severe coughing fits starting nearly 2 weeks later and lasting for up to 1 month; gasping for breath at the end of a coughing fit, causing the characteristic whoop.*

This childhood disease is spread by coughs and sneezes and is highly infectious during the early stages. It starts with the symptoms of a normal cold, followed 2 weeks later by violent, uncontrollable bouts of coughing, which frequently end in vomiting. Because the child cannot breathe in during these spasms, they may feel as though they are suffocating, and the typical 'whooping sound' is extremely distressing. In small babies, oxygen deprivation can become a real hazard. The coughing can also do permanent damage to the lungs. Home remedies can, however, speed recovery.

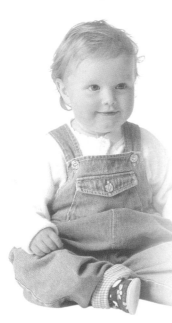

**BELOW** Whooping cough is a serious illness, but children can easily be immunized against it.

## ✚ CONVENTIONAL MEDICINE

If your child has been in contact with whooping cough and has not been immunized, then you should be on the lookout for symptoms, as it can only be treated during the first stage, before the coughing fits start. Treatment is with antibiotics.

## AROMATHERAPY

- Frankincense *(Boswellia sacra)*
- Lavender *(Lavandula angustifolia)*
- Sandalwood *(Santalum album)*

Frankincense and lavender are calming, slowing and deepen the breathing. Sandalwood is antispasmodic, calming and soothing.
**APPLICATION** Burn these oils in the sickroom, or massage the chest and back with them.

## HOMEOPATHIC REMEDIES

This is a serious condition and requires medical assessment.
- Drosera 6c

For deep spasms of coughing that start in the larynx, retching and vomiting. Worse at night, for lying down. Better for cold drinks.

♋ **Ipecacuanha 6c**

For spasmodic cough, suffocating, wheezing. Chest feels full of phlegm, but cannot cough it up. Constant feeling of nausea. Nosebleeds with cough.

♋ **Cuprum metallicum 6c**

For violent, spasmodic cough with vomiting. Better for drinking water. Tight feeling in chest.

DOSAGE 1 tablet every 4 hours. Maximum 2 weeks.

## HERBAL REMEDIES

Teas to help calm the child and reduce the violent coughing spasms can be used to support more orthodox remedies.

USE AND DOSAGE Combine a decoction of licorice and elecampane (1 tsp of each per cup) with an infusion of wild lettuce, thyme and camomile (1 tsp of each per cup), then give the child between 15ml/1tbsp and half a cup of the mix (diluted with water to make a whole cup), depending on age.

Use a chest rub of basil, hyssop and cypress oils (2 drops of each to 5ml/1tsp of almond oil).

Echinacea tablets help support the immune system (100–600mg daily in tablets, depending on age).

## NUTRITION

It is impossible to feed normal meals to a child with severe whooping cough. Give plenty of fluids – especially when the child is vomiting. Mixtures of warm apple juice, honey and water; pineapple and blackcurrant juice with warm water; warmed, mixed vegetable juices; warm ginger tea with honey; liquidized or clear soups, like vegetable or chicken broth; yeast extract drinks – all these will provide nutrients and are soothing. Try to avoid large amounts of milk during the first few days.

As the child begins to feel better, give small, light meals of scrambled egg; minced chicken with rice; fruit purées with cloves, cinnamon and honey; thin porridge with lots of honey; puréed potato and carrot, creamed with 1–2tbsp of very low-fat yogurt and a bit of nutmeg. Insist on giving regular intakes of liquid, even if just a dessertspoon at a time.

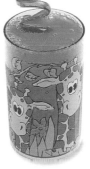

**BELOW** Encourage a child with whooping cough to take plenty of cold drinks, as these will ease deep coughing spasms.

**Caution**

Whooping cough is a serious illness, and although most children recover fully, complications can occur and medical care is essential, especially for those under the age of three.

**Prevention**

Avoid contact with other infected children, their siblings or parents. The risk of contracting this disease is greatly reduced by immunization, which is safe and effective.

# Scarlet fever

*Characterized by a fever; headache; vomiting; a thick white coat to the tongue with red spots; and a red rash (which is not itchy) on various parts of the body, often accompanied by flushed red cheeks.*

**S**carlet fever is nearly always the sequel to a bout of tonsillitis in children. They will often have a sore throat, pain on swallowing, a high temperature and inflamed tonsils, and if a rash appears 48 hours later on the neck, chest, stomach, arms and legs, then they are almost certainly suffering from scarlet fever. A hundred years ago this was the commonest cause of death in children over the age of one year – now it is rare. It is caused by a bacterial infection and usually lasts for about a week. Scarlet fever is infectious, so make sure that you keep children away from others who are suffering from it.

## Call the doctor

*If you suspect someone has scarlet fever.*

### Caution

*Scarlet fever can have serious complications, including rheumatic fever and inflammation of the kidneys, so consult a doctor if in doubt or if the condition persists. Always read pain-reliever packages carefully, and do not exceed the stated dose.*

## CONVENTIONAL MEDICINE

If you or your child show any symptoms of scarlet fever, contact your doctor. You can treat the fever with a simple pain reliever, but if your doctor confirms that you have scarlet fever, then you will probably need treatment with antibiotics.

**DOSAGE: ADULTS** 1–2 tablets of pain relievers at onset of fever, repeated every 4 hours; consult pack for details.

**DOSAGE: CHILDREN** Give regular doses of liquid pain reliever; consult pack, or follow medical advice.

## HOMEOPATHIC REMEDIES

Because of the serious complications of this disease, orthodox treatment is recommended for scarlet fever. Belladonna may, however, be used, together with orthodox medicine, to help relieve the symptoms.

### Belladonna 6c

For sudden red face and high temperature; could 'fry an egg' on the skin. Paleness around mouth, pupils dilated. Hallucinations.

**DOSAGE** 1 tablet every 2 hours for up to six doses, then every 4 hours as needed. Maximum 3 days.

## NUTRITION

A sore throat and tonsillitis will make eating painful and difficult, while a high temperature means that there will be a greatly increased need for fluid replacement (see *Fever* on p.16). Pineapple and pawpaw juices are of great value, as the natural enzymes that they contain are both soothing and extremely healing to the damaged and inflamed delicate membranes of the mouth and throat. Give plenty of vegetable soup made with masses of broccoli, leeks, onions, garlic and carrots, liquidized and presented warm in a cup. This will help boost the body's levels of the powerful antioxidant nutrients, which increase natural resistance.

PAWPAW

If antibiotics are administered, it is important to replace the natural bacteria in the gut, as these will be killed off by the medication. A twice-daily drink made of a carton of live yogurt, a dessertspoon of honey, a banana and 120ml/4fl oz of milk, blended into a smooth milkshake, should be given morning and evening.

**BELOW** Yogurt is ideal for a child suffering from scarlet fever, since it helps to renew the beneficial bacteria that are killed off by antibiotics.

## HERBAL REMEDIES

Certain herbs can alleviate the discomfort experienced during scarlet fever.

USE AND DOSAGE Try gargles containing 10–20 drops of either golden seal or myrrh tincture, or sage tea (2tsp per cup), to relieve a sore throat.

To help reduce fevers and ease discomfort, drink a tea containing a mix of catmint, camomile, elderflowers and boneset (½–2tsp of the mix per cup, depending on the child's age).

Echinacea tablets will help combat the infection: 100–600mg daily in tablets, depending on age.

# First aid

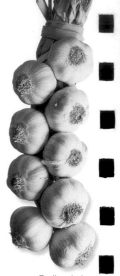

While it is important that you seek medical help for all emergencies, there are many less severe accidents and ailments that can safely be treated at home, using complementary first-aid remedies. Conventional medicine will often be the immediate standby when an accident occurs, but there are numerous herbal, homeo-pathic and aromatherapeutic remedies that can help to relieve the pain of a sting or burn, calm the person who has fainted or is suffering from motion sickness, and help wounds to heal after a bruise or bite has occurred. Nutrition, in the form of kitchen medicine, has a part to play, too – honey mixed with crushed garlic, for instance, makes an effective salve for cuts, while a traditional bread poultice will help to draw splinters to the surface.

**ABOVE** Garlic – being antibacterial and anti-fungal – has a role to play in first-aid treatment.

**LEFT** Many minor accidents can be treated at home, but if you are in doubt about the severity of a complaint, get medical help.

# Cuts

*Minor cuts do not usually require medical attention, because blood clots should quickly form and seal them, but they should be carefully cleaned and covered with a plaster or clean dressing when the bleeding stops.*

## KITCHEN MEDICINE

A heaped teaspoon of salt in 600ml/1pt of warm water makes a good emergency disinfectant. A compress made from a clean cloth soaked in 600ml/1pt of cold water and 10ml/2tsp of vinegar is also effective. To encourage healing, crushed garlic mixed with honey and then spread thinly on a piece of clean gauze makes a great salve.

**BELOW** Echinacea will help to prevent infection following a cut.

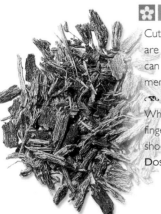

## ✚ CONVENTIONAL MEDICINE

Apply direct pressure over the cut for 10 minutes with a clean, dry cloth. If there is something stuck in the wound, such as glass, do not remove it, but apply pressure around it and seek medical advice. Raise the affected part of the body above chest level. If the cut is still bleeding after 10 minutes, reapply the dressing for a further 10 minutes. If the bleeding continues, apply pressure again and seek medical advice.

## HERBAL REMEDIES

After cleaning the cut with marigold infusion, apply creams or ointments containing marigold, chickweed, St John's wort, echinacea or camomile.

Emergency poultices can be made from crushed self-heal, woundwort, cranesbill, herb robert, agrimony or shepherd's purse.

## ◔ AROMATHERAPY

The most relevant oils are lavender and tea tree. Clean the cut area with a bowl of warm water containing 5 drops of either oil.

## ❋ HOMEOPATHIC REMEDIES

Cuts should be cleaned with water. Check that you are immunized against tetanus. Hypercal solution can be used to clean the wound, or hypercal ointment used under a clean dressing.

 Hypericum 30c
When injury is a puncture wound or injury to a fingertip that is rich in nerves. Pains often sharp and shooting.

**DOSAGE** 1 tablet every 4 hours. Maximum 3 days.

# Bruises

*Bruises are the visible sign of bleeding occurring beneath the skin, generally resulting either from pressure or from a blow. They usually change colour over a period of several days, depending on the amount of blood below the skin.*

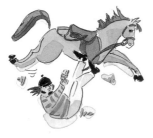

### CONVENTIONAL MEDICINE

Apply an ice pack as soon as possible after the injury to reduce the swelling and bruising. Take a pain reliever such as paracetamol or ibuprofen.

### HERBAL REMEDIES

Apply comfrey, chickweed or arnica creams or lotions (but do not use arnica if the skin is broken); a cold compress soaked in sanicle, rue or St John's wort infusion; or a crushed cabbage leaf (held in place with a sticking plaster if necessary).

## KITCHEN MEDICINE

Pineapple juice and ice packs (see *Black Eyes opposite*) are the best kitchen medicine there is for bruises. Massaging the bruised area with a little extra-virgin olive oil will disperse the bruise, and the vitamin E that penetrates the skin is an additional aid to healing.

### HOMEOPATHIC REMEDIES

**Arnica 30c**
The main remedy for bruises and also helpful in treating muscle aches after sport. Probably the first remedy to try. Very useful if the person does not want help and says they are okay, even when obviously they are not. Also good after surgery.

**Bellis perennis 30c**
For bruising that is deeper and for very sore muscles.

**Ledum 30c**
For very dark bruising. Area feels cold and is better for a cold compress.

**DOSAGE** 1 tablet every 2 hours for six doses, then three times daily. Maximum 5 days.

### AROMATHERAPY

Put 4 drops of lavender and camomile (2 drops of each) into a bowl of hot water and 2 drops of each into a bowl of cold water. Soak a facecloth in each bowl, then apply alternately to the bruised area — put the hot cloth on and, when that is cool, replace with the cold one; then repeat the process.

# Black eyes

*A black eye is the result of severe bruising of the eye socket and lids. It is internal bleeding that results in the swelling and the skin turning black or dark blue. Sadly, most black eyes are sustained through accident or anger.*

## CONVENTIONAL MEDICINE

Apply an ice pack as soon as possible after the injury to reduce the swelling and bruising. Take a pain reliever such as paracetamol or ibuprofen.

## HERBAL REMEDIES

Apply fresh *Aloe vera* sap or mashed plantain leaves; a cold compress soaked in rue or comfrey infusion.

## AROMATHERAPY

Put 1 drop of camomile into 10ml/2tsp of ice-cold water, soak a cottonwool pad, then apply to the affected area.

## HOMEOPATHIC REMEDIES

A couple of remedies will be effective in helping to treat black eyes.

### Aconite 30c

Give immediately for the 'shock' of the blow (can also be given for any sudden injury). One or two doses only, over 15 minutes.

### Ledum 30c

For a black eye that is generally better for cold compresses. The skin around the eye is usually swollen.

DOSAGE 1 tablet taken every 30 minutes for six doses, then repeat the dose every 2–4 hours. Maximum 12 doses.

### KITCHEN MEDICINE

The best kitchen medicine is not the old-fashioned remedy of a raw steak, but to drink copious amounts of pineapple juice – preferably before the injury (if you're a boxer); but even after the event the enzymes in pineapple juice speed up the rate at which the blood causing the black eye dissolves, so that it will heal more quickly. A clean tea towel filled with crushed ice and placed over the area hastens the healing.

### Caution

*Two black eyes after a blow to the head may be the sign of a skull fracture – seek urgent medical advice.*

# Bites

*If the skin is punctured – whether by an animal or human bite – you will need to check your anti-tetanus vaccination, but bites should always be seen by a doctor as soon as possible. Rinse the bitten area with copious amounts of water.*

**BELOW** *Aloe vera* sap is soothing and prevents infection.

## CONVENTIONAL MEDICINE

A bite from any animal (including a human bite) is highly vulnerable to infection, as all animals have germs in their mouths. After cleaning the wound carefully with soap and water, dry and then cover it with a plaster or a small sterile dressing, then seek medical attention.

## HERBAL REMEDIES

For insect bites, apply fresh *Aloe vera* sap; diluted lavender or tea-tree oil (5 drops in 5ml/1tsp of water); fresh lemon balm or plantain leaves.

Bathe with marigold or echinacea tea, if the bite becomes infected.

## HOMEOPATHIC REMEDIES

Hypercal tincture or lotion can be applied to the skin and may be soothing.

**Ledum 30c**

For insect bites with a lot of swelling. Discomfort eased when bathing in cold water or a cold compress applied. May prevent mosquito bites in people who are often bitten (for prevention: 1 tablet daily for a maximum of 14 days). Also useful in animal bites.

**Apis 30c**

For burning of surrounding area. Swelling often marked. Worse for heat.

**DOSAGE** 1 tablet every 30 minutes (every 15 minutes for a severe reaction). Maximum six doses.

## AROMATHERAPY

Put a neat drop of lavender directly onto the area of skin affected by the bite.

### KITCHEN MEDICINE

A real old wives' remedy if you are out in the countryside is to chew up a mouthful of plantain leaves and apply the resulting paste to the wound. Flea bites should be rubbed with a slice of raw onion; mosquito bites with the cut end of a clove of garlic.

# Stings

*Stings, by insects and marine animals, vary in strength and seriousness, but often result in localized pain, reddening and swelling, and sometimes in nausea, fainting and breathing problems.*

BEES

## CONVENTIONAL MEDICINE

If the sting is visible, remove it with tweezers. Apply a cold compress. Use calamine or antihistamine to reduce the itch, and apply insect repellent to prevent further bites.

## HERBAL REMEDIES

Apply a fresh slice of onion to bee and wasp stings; sage or marigold cream; crushed plantain leaves.

Bathe the area with sage or marigold infusions, after removing any remaining sting.

## AROMATHERAPY

Remove the sting if possible, then put 1 drop of neat lavender on the affected area, repeating the treatment if necessary following a plant sting (e.g. from a nettle).

## HOMEOPATHIC REMEDIES

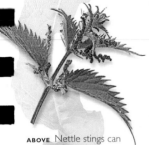

**ABOVE** Nettle stings can be relieved by rubbing with a dock leaf.

 Ledum 30c

For insect stings where there is a lot of swelling. Discomfort eased when bathing affected area in cold water or a cold compress is applied.

 Apis 30c

For burning and stinging of surrounding area. Swelling often marked. Worse for heat. Good treatment for bee and wasp stings.

**DOSAGE** 1 tablet every 30 minutes (every 15 minutes for a severe reaction). Maximum six doses.

### KITCHEN MEDICINE

For wasp stings, make a paste of salt and vinegar, then spread over the affected area. For bee stings, use baking powder or sodium bicarbonate, mixed to a smooth paste – making sure that you remove the sting.

The traditional remedy for stinging nettle burns is the dock leaf, but an ordinary used teabag dipped in iced water can be equally soothing; as can a cup of nettle tea.

### Caution

*Wasps are the most likely to sting the inside of your mouth or throat. Sucking ice cubes will relieve the swelling, but at the slightest sign of breathing difficulties, rush to your nearest hospital.*

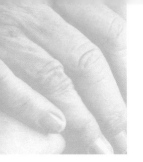

# Burns

*Burns are often accompanied by shock. Never, never use
butter or oil on them. For small areas, run the affected part
under cold water, or immerse the burned area until the pain
diminishes – usually for at least 10–15 minutes.*

## Caution

*Severe burns need
urgent hospital
treatment.*

## CONVENTIONAL MEDICINE

Run cold water onto the burned skin until the
burning sensation stops. Remove burned clothing,
unless it is stuck to the burn. Cover with clean, non-
fluffy material, such as a clean pillowcase, a plastic
bag or clingfilm. If the burn is extensive, located on
the face or anywhere near the mouth, seek immediate medical advice.

## HOMEOPATHIC REMEDIES

For minor burns, cool the area with cold water.
Chemical burns need specialist treatment.

**Arnica 30c**
Initial remedy to take after any trauma.
**DOSAGE** 1 tablet every 15 minutes for four doses.
Then try the following:

**Cantharis 30c**
For burn that feels as if it is raw, with severe pains.
Better for cold being applied. May have blistering.
**DOSAGE** 1 tablet every 15 minutes for six doses,
then every 4 hours. Maximum 12 doses.

## KITCHEN MEDICINE

Anyone who has
suffered from sunburn
or serious burns, to an
area greater than your
hand can readily cover,
should be given plenty
of fluids to drink in
order to prevent
dehydration.

## HERBAL REMEDIES

For minor burns, apply a compress soaked in cool
chickweed, St John's wort, marigold or plantain infusion; a little infused oil of St John's wort, after first
cooling the area under a running tap; fresh sap
from an *Aloe vera* plant; or slippery-elm powder
that has been mixed with a little milk or water to
form a paste.

## AROMATHERAPY

First run the burn under freezing cold water, then
immediately put some neat lavender oil on it.

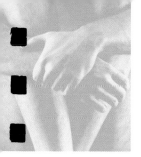

# Sunburn

*Sunburn is caused by ultraviolet rays and your susceptibility depends on your colouring and the amount of pigment in your skin. It is difficult to believe there is anyone unaware of the links between excessive sun exposure and skin cancer.*

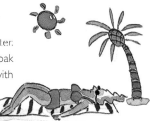

## CONVENTIONAL MEDICINE

Find some shade and drink plenty of cold water. Sponge the sunburned skin with cold water or soak it in a cold bath. Mild burns can be soothed with calamine or an after-sun preparation.

## HERBAL REMEDIES

Apply infused St John's wort oil with a few drops of lavender oil; fresh *Aloe vera* sap or ointment; evening primrose or borage cream when the burn starts to heal.

Drink an infusion of lime flowers, elderflowers and yarrow to encourage sweating.

## HOMEOPATHIC REMEDIES

**Belladonna 6c**

For red face, very hot to touch, 'could fry an egg on it'. Throbbing headache, worse for light and noise. May have high fever and dilated pupils.

**Glonoine 6c**

For bursting headache with waves of pulsating pain. Worse during hours of sun, even if not directly exposed to it. Worse for moving. Face may be flushed or pale.

**DOSAGE** 1 tablet every half hour for six doses, then every 4 hours. Maximum 4 days.

## AROMATHERAPY

Add peppermint or lavender to a cool bath or, if the sunburn is quite bad, drip lavender oil on neat after a cool bath, repeating every 2–3 hours if necessary. If the sunburned area is too tender to touch, apply the oils in a water spray. After a little too much sun, add the oils to aftersun lotion.

### KITCHEN MEDICINE

Relieve mild to moderate sunburn by putting three or four camomile teabags into a tepid bath and soaking for 15 minutes. A mixture of one part olive oil and two parts cider vinegar, rubbed gently into the affected skin, will also help.

### Call the doctor

*For cases of severe sunburn with blisters.*

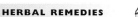

# Sprains

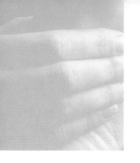

SEAWEED

*A sprain occurs when the ligaments surrounding and supporting a joint are either overstretched or torn, most commonly in the ankle or wrist.*

## KITCHEN MEDICINE

An ice pack applied to the injury (see *Nosebleeds on p.182*) will help. Soothing baths bring great relief: add a heaped tablespoon of mustard powder or a cup of Epsom salts. A bucket of seawater added to a hot bath, or a handful of seaweed, can also be extremely healing for sprains.

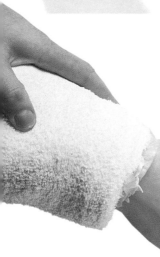

## ✚ CONVENTIONAL MEDICINE

Apply an ice pack or cold compress as soon as possible to reduce swelling and bruising. Put on a bandage or tubigrip to provide gentle, even pressure. Avoid using the sprained joint, and raise it in a sling or on a foot stool. Take a pain reliever.

## ❋ HOMEOPATHIC REMEDIES

### ⌁ Arnica 30c

Take for the initial bruising.

**DOSAGE** 1 tablet every 15 minutes for four doses. Continue if bruising is the main problem, at a dose of 1 tablet twice daily. Maximum 5 days.

### ⌁ Ledum 6c

For sprains, particularly of the ankle, when it is black with bruising and is better for cold compresses.

### ⌁ Rhus toxicodendron 6c

Pain worse on initial movement, improves as joint is 'warmed up' by movement. Worse in the morning when the joint seems stiff. Better during the day and for warm weather. Person may be restless.

**DOSAGE** 1 tablet three times daily. Maximum 2 weeks.

## ◪ HERBAL REMEDIES

Use crushed comfrey or cabbage leaves as a poultice.

Apply arnica, comfrey or marigold creams, with a few drops of lavender or thyme oil added; or use a compress soaked in an infusion or diluted tincture.

Soak the affected area with an ice pack and a hot rosemary infusion: use a foot bath or compress.

## ◔ AROMATHERAPY

Ice the sprain to reduce any swelling, then massage the whole area using ginger, lavender and camomile.

# Fractures

*A fracture is a broken or cracked bone, which is generally caused either by direct force (such as a blow or a kick) or by means of indirect force, when the bone breaks at some distance from the actual point of force.*

## CONVENTIONAL MEDICINE

Keep the fractured bone still. Discourage the injured person from drinking or eating anything, in case surgery is necessary. Support the injured part with your hands without moving it. If possible, make a sling to hold a broken arm against the body; a broken leg can be strapped to the other leg for support. Seek urgent medical attention.

## HOMEOPATHIC REMEDIES

Homeopathic remedies may assist orthodox medical treatment.

**Arnica 30c**
Take this remedy first, for the associated bruising.
DOSAGE 1 tablet every 2 hours for six doses.

**Symphytum 6c** (also called boneset/boneknit)
May help with the joining up of the broken bones. Also used when the fracture is slow to mend.

**Calcarea phosphorica 6c**
Use if symphytum does not help.
DOSAGE 1 tablet twice daily. Maximum 14 days.

## HERBAL REMEDIES

Freshly pulped comfrey leaves used as a poultice will be beneficial for minor cracks or broken toes.

Drink an infusion of horsetail, alfalfa and comfrey to encourage healing of the fracture.

## AROMATHERAPY

You cannot massage the fracture itself, so you need to work on the corresponding area (i.e. if the wrist is fractured, massage the ankle on the same side; for the shoulder, work the hip). Choose a soothing essential oil *(see Stress on p.36).*

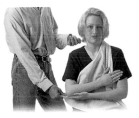

To make a sling, lay a triangular bandage with the point beyond the elbow of the injured arm.

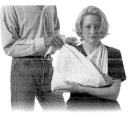

Lift the lower end of the bandage over the injured arm while the patient supports it.

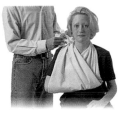

Tie the end to the neck end by the collarbone. Tuck in (or pin) the bandage by the elbow.

# Nosebleeds

*Nosebleeds may be caused either by illness or by a blow; they may also be occasioned by rupturing the nasal blood vessels, but sometimes they simply occur spontaneously for no apparent reason.*

## KITCHEN MEDICINE

The best remedy is in your refrigerator – crush a few cubes of ice and wrap them in a clean handkerchief. Place this ice pack over the top of the nose and apply pressure with the thumb and forefinger on each side for at least 5–6 minutes. If the bleeding persists, put 10ml/2tsp of cider vinegar into a glass of tepid water, tip the head back and use a dropper to trickle the mixture into each nostril.

## ✚ CONVENTIONAL MEDICINE

Sit down, leaning forwards. Breathing through the mouth, pinch the soft part of the nose below the bridge. Avoid sniffing, swallowing, coughing or spitting, which might provoke further bleeding. Use a handkerchief or cloth to mop up the blood. Release the pressure after 10 minutes. If bleeding continues, reapply pressure for another 10 minutes. After 30 minutes, if the bleeding has not stopped, seek medical advice. If the bleeding does stop, you should rest quietly for several hours and avoid sniffing or blowing. If a broken nose is suspected, keep holding the nose and get medical help.

## ✿ HOMEOPATHIC REMEDIES

For persistent nosebleeds, consult your doctor.
### ❧ Arnica 30c
For nosebleeds resulting from a blow to the nose. This helps stop the bleeding.
### ❧ Phosphorus 30c
Often used in children. For nosebleeds for no apparent reason. Bright red blood, and nosebleeds when blowing the nose.
**DOSAGE** 1 tablet every 15 minutes. Maximum six doses.

## HERBAL REMEDIES

A traditional and effective herbal remedy is simply to insert a yarrow leaf in the affected nostril and then pinch the nose together gently until a blood clot forms.

Insert a small cotton swab soaked in shepherd's purse, witch hazel, lady's mantle, agrimony or yarrow tincture into the nostril.

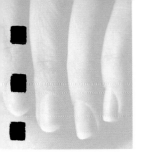

# Splinters

*Splinters are generally small pieces of wood or thorn that get embedded in the skin and may cause infection. Soak the affected area in hot, very soapy water before squeezing the splinter out or removing it with a sterilized needle or tweezers.*

## CONVENTIONAL MEDICINE

If possible, remove the splinter with tweezers. If the splinter is deeply embedded or difficult to remove, seek medical advice. Clean the area around the splinter with soap and warm water. Check that your tetanus immunization is up to date.

## HERBAL REMEDIES

Use a little chickweed, marsh-mallow or slippery-elm ointment to help draw stubborn splinters: apply the ointment, cover with a small bandage and leave for a few hours before extracting the splinter with tweezers or a clean needle.

## AROMATHERAPY

Remove the splinter with tweezers or a sterilized needle, then apply 1 drop of neat lavender oil to the site.

## HOMEOPATHIC REMEDIES

Remove the splinter if at all possible. Watch for signs of infection.

### Silicea 6c

Reputed to expel foreign material from the body. Care should be taken, as it may also aid expulsion of pins or screws used to keep a fracture in place! Has been known to irritate dental fillings. If this occurs, stop.

**Dosage** 1 tablet twice daily. Maximum 14 days.

**RIGHT**
Marsh mallow ointment helps draw out splinters.

### KITCHEN MEDICINE

For stubborn and difficult splinters, cover the area with a hot bread poultice, which will help to draw the splinter to the surface. Make this by putting three or four slices of bread (white, brown or wholemeal – it makes no real difference) into a sieve. Pour over boiling water, then mash with a wooden spoon until you have a thick, hot paste. Make sure that the temperature is not too hot before applying. For really stubborn splinters, especially underneath finger- or toenails, you may need several applications.

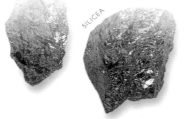

SILICEA

# Motion sickness

*Any form of motion can cause the nausea, vomiting and dizziness that we know as motion sickness. It is much more common in children, but adults too can suffer. There is a link between severe motion sickness in children and adult migraine.*

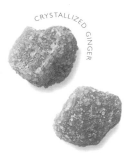

CRYSTALLIZED GINGER

**ABOVE** Ginger in all its forms can alleviate nausea and sickness.

## KITCHEN MEDICINE

Ginger is the king of kitchen remedies, but for maximum benefit you need to administer it before the sickness starts. Fill a thermos flask with ginger tea and, after your pre-travel mugful, sip a small cup every hour. For children, buy crystallized ginger, cut it into small cubes, dust liberally with icing sugar and give to the young-ster to nibble on every half-hour.

## CONVENTIONAL MEDICINE

Symptoms can be prevented by lying flat with closed eyes. Try to avoid reading while moving. If possible, get out of the vehicle or take a break from travelling.

## HOMEOPATHIC REMEDIES

Homeopathic motion-sickness pills (a combination of remedies) are available from some chemists.

**Cocculus 30c**

For nausea and giddiness at even the thought of food. Lots of saliva. Giddiness better for lying down. Worse for watching moving objects, for loss of sleep, light and noise.

**Tabacum 30c**

For person convinced they will die of nausea. Pale with cold sweats. Worse for opening eyes and smell of tobacco. Better in fresh cold air (on deck).

**Petroleum 30c**

For nausea that is worse for sitting up, noise. Better for eating. Lots of saliva.

**DOSAGE** 1 tablet every 30 minutes until improved. Maximum six doses.

## HERBAL REMEDIES

Drink a cup of camomile, black horehound, lemon balm or meadowsweet as tea, or use 2–3 drops of tincture on the tongue at regular intervals.

## AROMATHERAPY

Put a couple of drops of ginger or peppermint oil on a handkerchief; or rub a lotion containing them into the hands; alternatively, massage the upper abdomen with the essential oils.

# Fainting

*Fainting is caused by a temporary reduction in the supply of blood to the brain. It may be due to a shock, fear or exhaustion, missed meals, an over-hot atmosphere or standing still for too long.*

## CONVENTIONAL MEDICINE

Encourage the person to lie down with their legs raised about 15cm/6in, until they feel completely better. Check for injuries, such as bruising or cuts. Make a note of the events that occurred before, during and after the faint (useful information for the doctor) and encourage the patient to have a medical check-up.

## HOMEOPATHIC REMEDIES

**Carbo vegetabilis 6c**
For chilly person, who collapses with cold sweats. Wants air and to be fanned. Fainting from too much food.

**Phosphorus 6c**
For open, lively and artistic person. Sympathetic and sensitive to external impressions. Fainting from hunger.

**Ignatia 6c**
For fainting from emotional shock. Person is grief-stricken, sighing. Intolerant of tobacco. Lump in throat, as if about to cry.
**DOSAGE** 1 tablet every 10 minutes. Maximum 12 tablets. Crush tablet and place powder on the tongue.

## AROMATHERAPY

Loosen all clothing, make sure that the person is comfortable, then waft under their nose some rosemary, peppermint or basil oil.

## HERBAL REMEDIES

Sniff camphor or tea-tree oil.
    Drink camomile or betony tea to help recovery, once consciousness is regained.

### KITCHEN MEDICINE

A cup of hot green or Indian tea sweetened with honey should be sipped once the fainting has passed. And inhaling the aroma from a small piece of crushed horseradish is a good substitute for old-fashioned smelling salts.

ROSEMARY

# Herbal remedies
## basic methods

**A**lthough it is possible to buy many herbal remedies commercially, it is often cheaper to make your own at home and create just the amount you need. All quantities given throughout the herbal sections refer to dried herbs, rather than fresh.

### MAKING A COMPRESS

A compress (either hot or cold) is an effective way of applying a herbal remedy directly to the site of an inflammation or skin wound in order to speed up the healing process. Soak a clean linen or cotton cloth, or a pad of cottonwool, in a hot infusion or decoction (see below and p.187). Apply to the affected skin as hot as is bearable, either changing it as it cools down or covering it with plastic or waxed paper, and then with a hot-water bottle, to maintain its temperature. Prepare a cold compress in the same way, but allow it to cool before applying directly to the skin.

### MAKING A POULTICE

A poultice consists of a pulp made directly of herbs. It is often used to draw pus out of the skin. Mix dried herbs with a little hot water until you have a paste; or use the mushy herbs left over from a hot infusion or decoction (see below and p.187); or process fresh herbs in a food mixer. Sandwich the paste between two layers of gauze, then apply to the affected skin as hot as is bearable, changing it or placing a hot-water bottle on top, as for a compress.

### MAKING AN INFUSION

Infusions are the most versatile method of taking herbal remedies, since you can drink them as teas or tisanes (hot or cold, sweetened with a little honey, if desired); use them as a mouth-wash, gargle or eyebath (simmered to sterilize, then cooled); or add them to the bath. They are made from the flowers or leaves of the plant, which readily release their active ingredients. Warm a china or glass teapot, then add the dried herb, breaking it into small pieces if necessary. Cover with near-boiling water. Allow 1–2tsp of the herb for each cup of water. Steep for 5–10 minutes, then strain and drink. Make fresh infusions each day.

### MAKING A DECOCTION

Decoctions are similar to infusions, and are used in much the same way, but involve boiling the herb to release its active ingredients. This enables woody stems, roots, bark, berries and seeds to be used. Chop or crush the herb into an enamel, stainless-steel or glass-lidded pan (never aluminium). Cover with cold water. Allow 1½ cups of water to ½–1tsp of herb. Bring to the boil and simmer for 10–15 minutes or until the volume is reduced by one-third. Strain and use while still hot. It is preferable to make fresh decoctions daily.

### MAKING A TINCTURE

Tinctures are alcohol preparations. The alcohol dissolves most of the herb's useful ingredients and preserves the preparation. Tinctures are stronger than infusions or decoctions and are best diluted with a little water. Place some chopped or powdered herb in a container with a tightly fitting lid. Use a ratio of 1 part herb to 5 parts liquid (e.g. 200g to 1l, or 1lb to 5pt). Pour over a water/alcohol mix, made by diluting a bottle of vodka with half its amount of water. Leave for 2 weeks, shaking regularly, then strain through a muslin cloth, squeezing it out well. Pour into dark glass bottles and keep well stoppered in a cool, dark place. The dosage is generally 5ml/1tsp three times a day.

### MAKING A SUGAR SYRUP

Syrups are concentrated sugar preparations, which help preserve infusions and decoctions and mask the unpalatable taste of some herbs. They can make cough mixtures and herbal brews more acceptable to children. Bring some of your selected infusion or decoction to the boil with honey or sugar, using the ratio 500ml liquid to 500g honey or sugar (1pt to 1lb). When the mixture turns syrupy, store until required in a corked bottle (not a screwtop one).

# Herbs mentioned
# with botanical names

| COMMON NAME | Botanical name |
|---|---|
| AGNUS-CASTUS | Vitex agnus-castus |
| AGRIMONY | Agrimonia eupatoria |
| ALFALFA | Medicago sativa |
| ALOE VERA | Aloe vera |
| AMERICAN GINSENG | Panax quinquefolius |
| ANGELICA | Angelica archangelica |
| ANISE | Pimpinella anisum |
| ARNICA | Arnica montana |
| ASTRAGALUS | Astragalus membranaceus |
| BASIL | Ocimum basilicum |
| BAYBERRY | Myrica cerifera |
| BEARBERRY | Arctostaphylos uva-ursi |
| BENZOIN | Styrax benzoin |
| (FRIAR'S BALSAM — compound tincture of benzoin) | |
| BETONY | Stachys officinalis |
| BILBERRY | Vaccinium myrtillus |
| BIRCH | Betula pendula |
| BISTORT | Polygonum bistorta |
| BITTER ORANGE | Citrus aurantium |
| BLACK COHOSH | Cimicifuga racemosa |
| BLACK HAW | Viburnum prunifolium |
| BLACK HOREHOUND | Ballota nigra |
| BLUE COHOSH | Caulophyllum thalictroides |
| BLUE FLAG | Iris versicolor |
| BOGBEAN | Menyanthes trifoliata |
| BONESET | Eupatorium perfoliatum |
| BORAGE | Borago officinalis |
| BUCHU | Agathosma crenulata |
| BUCKWHEAT | Fagopyrum esculentum (now known as Polygonum fagopyrum) |
| BURDOCK | Arctium lappa |
| CABBAGE | Brassica oleracea |
| CADE OIL | Eucalyptus globulus |
| CALIFORNIAN POPPY | Eschscholzia californica |
| CAMOMILE | Matricaria recutita |
| CARAWAY | Carum carvi |
| CARDAMOM | Elettaria cardamomum |
| CASCARA SAGRADA | Rhamnus purshianus |
| CATMINT | Nepeta cataria |
| CAYENNE | Capsicum frutescens |
| CENTAURY | Centaurium erythraea |
| CHICKWEED | Stellaria media |
| CHILLI | Capsicum anuum |

| COMMON NAME | Botanical name |
|---|---|
| CHINESE FIGWORT (XUAN SHEN) | Scrophularia ningpoensis |
| CINNAMON | Cinnamomum zeylanicum |
| CLEAVERS | Galium aparine |
| CLOVE | Syzgium aromaticum |
| CODONOPSIS | Codonopsis tangstien |
| COFFEE | Coffea arabica |
| COLA | Cola nitida |
| COLTSFOOT | Tussilago farfara |
| COMFREY | Symphytum officinale |
| COMMON PLANTAIN | Plantago major |
| CORIANDER | Coriandrum sativum |
| CORNSILK | Zea mays |
| COUCHGRASS | Elymus repens |
| COWSLIP | Primula veris |
| CRAMP BARK | Viburnum opulus |
| CRANBERRY | Vaccinium oxycoccos |
| CRANESBILL | Geranium spp. |
| CYPRESS | Cupressus sempervirens |
| DAMIANA | Turnera diffusa |
| DANDELION | Taraxacum officinale |
| DANG GUI | Angelica polyphorma var. sinensis |
| DEVIL'S CLAW | Harpagophytum procumbens |
| DILL | Anethum graveolens |
| DOCK | Rumex obtusifolius |
| ECHINACEA | Echinacea spp. |
| ELDER | Sambucus nigra |
| ELECAMPANE | Inula helenium |
| EPHEDRA | Ephedra distachya |
| EUCALYPTUS | Eucalyptus globulus |
| EVENING PRIMROSE | Oenothera biennis |
| EYEBRIGHT | Euphrasia officinalis |
| FENNEL | Foeniculum vulgare |
| FENUGREEK | Trigonella foenum graecum |
| FEVERFEW | Tanacetum parthienium |
| FORSYTHIA | Forsythia suspensa |
| FRINGE TREE | Chionanthus virginicus |
| FUMITORY | Fumaria officinalis |
| GALANGAL | Alpinia officinarum |
| GARLIC | Allium sativa |
| GENTIAN | Gentiana lutea |
| GINGER | Zingiber officinale |

| COMMON NAME | Botanical name | COMMON NAME | Botanical name |
|---|---|---|---|
| GINKGO | Ginkgo biloba | PAU D'ARCO | Tabebuia impetiginosa |
| GINSENG | Panax ginseng | PAWPAW | Carica papaya |
| GOLDEN SEAL | Hydrastis canadensis | PEPPERMINT | Mentha x piperita |
| GOTU KOLA | Centella asiatica | PILEWORT | Ranunculus ficaria |
| GREATER CELANDINE | Chelidonium majus | PINE | Pinus sylvestris |
| GROUND IVY | Glechoma hederacea | POPLAR | Populus alba |
| GUARANA | Paullinia cupana | PRICKLY ASH | Zanthoxylum americanum |
| HEARTSEASE | Viola tricolor | RASPBERRY | Rubus idaeus |
| HELONIAS | Chamaelirium luteum | RED CLOVER | Trifolium pratense |
| HERB ROBERT | Geranium robertianum | REISHI | Ganoderma lucidum |
| HE SHOU WU/FO TI | Polygonum multiflorum | RIBWORT PLANTAIN | Plantago lanceolata |
| HOLY THISTLE | Cnicus benedictus | ROSE | Rosa spp. |
| HOPS | Humulus lupulus | ROSEMARY | Rosmarinus officinalis |
| HORSE CHESTNUT | Aesculus hippocastanum | SAGE | Salvia officinalis |
| HORSERADISH | Armoracia rusticana | ST JOHN'S WORT | Hypericum perforatum |
| HORSETAIL | Equisetum arvense | SANDALWOOD | Santalum album |
| HOUSE LEEK | Sempervivum tectorum | SANICLE | Sanicula europaea |
| HYSSOP | Hyssopus officinalis | SELF-HEAL | Prunella vulgaris |
| IRISH MOSS | Chondrus crispus | SENNA | Senna alexandrina |
| ISPAGHULA | Plantago psyllium | SHEPHERD'S PURSE | Capsella bursa-pastoris |
| JASMINE | Jasminum officinale | SHIITAKE MUSHROOM | Lentinus edodes |
| JUNIPER | Juniperus communis | SIBERIAN GINSENG | Eleutherococcus senticosus |
| KELP | Fucus versiculosus | SILVERWEED | Potentilla anserina |
| KOREAN GINSENG | see Ginseng | SKULLCAP | Scutellaria lateriflora |
| LADY'S MANTLE | Alchemilla vulgaris | SLIPPERY ELM | Ulmus rubra |
| LAVENDER | Lavandula angustifolia | SOAPWORT | Saponaria oficinalis |
| LEMON BALM | Melissa officinalis | STINGING NETTLE | Urtica dioica |
| LICORICE | Glycyrrhiza glabra | SWEET SUMACH | Rhus aromatica |
| LIFE ROOT | Senecio aureus | TANGERINE | Citrus reticulata |
| LIME FLOWERS | Tilia cordata | TANSY | Tanacetum vulgare |
| LOBELIA | Lobelia inflata | TEA | Camellia sinensis |
| LOVAGE | Levisticum officinale | TEA TREE | Melaleuca alternifolia |
| MALABAR TAMARIND | Garcinia cambogia | THUJA | Thuja occidentalis |
| MARIGOLD | Calendula officinalis | THYME | Thymus vulgaris |
| MARJORAM | Origanum majorana | TORMENTIL | Potentilla erecta |
| MARSH CUDWEED | Gnaphthalium uliginosum | TURNIP | Brassica 'Rapifero Group' |
| MARSH-MALLOW | Althaea officinalis | VALERIAN | Valeriana officinalis |
| MEADOWSWEET | Filipendula ulmaria | VERVAIN | Verbena officinalis |
| MELILOT | Melilotus officinalis | VIOLET | Viola odorata |
| MILK THISTLE | Silybum marianum (previously Carduus marianus) | WHITE HOREHOUND | Marrubium vulgare |
| | | WHITE WILLOW/ BLACK WILLOW | Salix alba/S. nigra |
| MOTHERWORT | Leonurus cardiaca | WILD CHERRY | Prunus serotina |
| MUGWORT | Artemisia vulgaris | WILD INDIGO | Baptisia tinctoria |
| MULLEIN | Verbascum thapsus | WILD LETTUCE | Lactuca virosa |
| MYRRH | Commiphora molmol | WILD YAM | Dioscorea villosa |
| NUTMEG | Myristica fragrans | WINTERGREEN | Gaultheria procumbens |
| OAK | Quercus robur | WITCH HAZEL | Hamamelis virginiana |
| OATS | Avena sativa | WORMWOOD | Artemisia absintheum |
| ONION | Allium cepa | WOUNDWORT | Stachys palustris |
| PARSLEY | Petroselinum crispum | YARROW | Achillea millefolium |
| PARSLEY PIERT | Aphanes arvensis | YELLOW DOCK | Rumex crispus |
| PASSIONFLOWER | Passiflora incarnata | | |

# Most useful herbal remedies

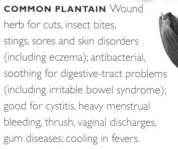

GARLIC

**AGRIMONY** Soothes digestive problems (including diarrhoea and food intolerance), cuts and grazes, skin problems, minor eye problems (e.g. conjunctivitis), sore throats and catarrh.

**ALOE VERA** Effective for skin problems, minor cuts and burns, insect bites, digestive problems; acts as an appetite stimulant and tonic.

**BETONY** Relaxing nervine for anxiety and stress, headaches, cuts and bruises, mouth and gum disorders, sore throats; encourages contractions in childbirth; acts as a digestive stimulant and as a circulatory tonic.

**CAMOMILE** Beneficial for digestive problems (including irritable bowel syndrome and indigestion), poor appetite, insomnia, nervous tension and anxiety, mouth inflammations and sore throats, minor eye problems, nasal catarrh, eczema and skin problems, asthma and hay fever; homeopathic dilutions for colic, restlessness and teething problems in babies and toddlers.

**COMMON PLANTAIN** Wound herb for cuts, insect bites, stings, sores and skin disorders (including eczema); antibacterial, soothing for digestive-tract problems (including irritable bowel syndrome); good for cystitis, heavy menstrual bleeding, thrush, vaginal discharges, gum diseases; cooling in fevers.

**ECHINACEA** Antibacterial, antiviral and antifungal for a range of infections (including colds/flu), for skin problems like athlete's foot and acne, sore throats, kidney infections.

**ELDER** The flowers are useful for catarrh, colds, flu, hay fever, fevers and inflammation; the leaves can be used in ointments for bruises and sores.

**GARLIC** Antibacterial, antifungal and antiseptic; lowers blood cholesterol levels and useful to combat candidiasis and respiratory infections; strengthens the immune system.

**GINGER** Warming for chills and colds; combats nausea and vomiting; calming for the digestive system (especially indigestion and flatulence); acts as a circulatory stimulant.

**LAVENDER** Sedative and cooling for migraines, headaches, insomnia and stress; good for digestive upsets (including indigestion); use externally on burns, grazes and sunburn.

GINGER

**LEMON BALM** Calming for digestive upsets and nervous problems; antidepressive; antibacterial — useful for infections and fevers; use externally to put on wounds, on insect bites and as an effective insect repellent.

**MARIGOLD** Good in creams for cuts, grazes, fungal infections, eczema and many other skin problems; acts as a digestive stimulant, and as a menstrual regulator; cooling in fevers; beneficial for gum disease and swollen glands.

**MARSH-MALLOW** Soothing for digestive inflammations and ulceration, urinary inflammations, coughs, catarrh, use externally for skin sores, boils, abscesses, and for drawing splinters and pus.

**MEADOWSWEET** Calming and antacid for digestive upsets (including gastritis and ulceration); good for arthritic and rheumatic disorders; antiseptic and cooling.

**ROSEMARY** Stimulating and restorative for nervous exhaustion and depression; beneficial for headaches, migraine, digestive problems (including gall-bladder problems, indigestion, etc.); use externally for arthritic and rheumatic pains.

**ST JOHN'S WORT** Antidepressive, sedative, restorative for the nervous system; useful in anxiety, nervous tension, depression, neuralgia, post-operative pain, period pain; antiseptic and soothing, so useful topically for burns, skin sores, cuts and grazes.

**TEA TREE** Antiseptic, antifungal; useful for all infections, including thrush, athlete's foot, ringworm, septicaemia, tooth and gum infections and abscesses, warts, cold sores, acne, insect stings and bites.

**THYME** Respiratory antiseptic and expectorant for coughs and bronchitis; acts as a digestive stimulant — warming for both chills and diarrhoea; the oil is antiseptic, for use as a wound herb and in cases of infection.

**VERVAIN** Relaxing nervine for depression and tension; acts as a digestive and liver stimulant; used in childbirth to ease labour pains; use topically for nerve pains (neuralgia)

**YARROW** Used in fevers and to dilate peripheral blood vessels; acts as a wound herb, digestive tonic and is helpful for both urinary and menstrual irregularities.

ROSEMARY

# Most useful conventional remedies

**ANTACIDS** Relieve indigestion; usually contain magnesium or aluminium salts. The latter (Aluminium hydroxide, Alu-Cap) may cause constipation; the former (e.g. Milk of Magnesia) may cause diarrhoea. Some preparations contain both aluminium and magnesium (e.g. Gaviscon, Mucogel, Maalox). Other mixtures contain dimethicone in order to relieve wind (e.g. Asilone, Simeco, Sovol).

**ANTIHISTAMINE** Tablets such as loratadine (Clarityn) or citirizine (Zirtek) help to relieve the symptoms of hay fever without causing drowsiness.

**BECLOMETHASONE DIPROPRIONATE** (Beconase) A nasal spray that relieves a long-standing problem with a blocked or dripping nose, such as occurs in hay fever. If the spray causes dryness and crusting, then seek medical advice for an alternative preparation.

**BENZOCAINE** (e.g. Dequacaine, Merocaine, Tyrozets) A local anaesthetic that is found in either lozenges or sprays; relieves the pain of sore throats.

**CALAMINE** Found in many treatments used to treat itching skin.

**CHLORPHENIRAMINE MALEATE TABLETS** (e.g. Piriton) Useful to prevent itching at night; not so useful during the day as it causes drowsiness. Also used to prevent jet lag and motion sickness.

**CIMETIDINE** (Tagamet) or **RANITIDINE** (Zantac) May help with indigestion that does not respond to an antacid. *Avoid in pregnancy.*

**CLOTRIMAZOLE** (Canestan) An antifungal treatment available as cream and pessaries; provides relief for thrush, although it may cause stinging (if so, seek medical advice).

**EMOLLIENTS** (e.g. E45 and oilatum) May alleviate dry skin; can be added to bath water or applied directly to the skin, and used for babies. Almond oil can help to soften ear wax prior to syringing.

**FLUCONAZOLE** (Diflucan One) Available as a single tablet, as an alternative to creams/pessaries to treat vaginal thrush. *Avoid in pregnancy.*

**HYDROCORTISONE ACETATE 1%**
A mild steroid cream, useful for skin irritation, such as mild eczema; can be used to stop tickly ears: apply gently to the ear canal with the little finger.

**IBUPROFEN** (e.g. Nurofen, Proflex or Reclofen) A painkiller, helpful where there is inflammation – e.g. sprains, backache or swollen joints. *Avoid if you have asthma or stomach ulcers. Avoid in pregnancy.*

**ISPAGHULA HUSK** (e.g. Fybogel) Useful for constipation that does not respond to dietary change/exercise. Children may prefer the taste of lactulose, which softens the faeces and takes a couple of days to work.

**MICONAZOLE** (Daktarin, Femeron) A spray for easy treatment of fungal skin infections, such as athlete's foot. Miconazole gel is available for treating oral thrush. *Avoid oral treatment in pregnancy.*

**PARACETAMOL** (e.g. Panadol or Hedex) A painkiller useful for treating headaches, sprains and fever. Many other tablets contain paracetamol with other drugs, such as codeine phosphate and caffeine, to enhance their effect. Be aware that codeine phosphate may cause constipation. *Avoid if you have liver problems.*

**POTASSIUM CITRATE** (e.g. Cymalon) Useful to relieve the symptoms of mild urine infection.

**RUBEFACIENT** (e.g. Deep Heat or Ralgex) Sprayed or rubbed onto the skin, it produces heat or cold and can ease a sprained joint/muscle ache.

## CHILDREN'S REMEDIES

**ALMOND OIL** Can help to soften cradle cap.

**CHLORPHENIRAMINE MALEATE LIQUID** (e.g. Piriton) Useful for treating itchy skin, particularly when it occurs at night

**DIMETHICONE** (e.g. Infacol) Can be used to treat infantile colic

Also **IBUPROFEN** (e.g. Junifen) and **PARACETAMOL** (e.g. Disprol, Calpol, Medinol, Infadrops), as above.

## SYMPTOMS THAT REQUIRE URGENT MEDICAL ATTENTION

- Temperature of more than 39.5°C/103°F
- Vomiting for more than 24 hours
- Difficulty rousing someone/ unconsciousness for more than 2 minutes
- Unexplained confused behaviour
- Not specifically unwell child, but possibly lethargic and floppy
- Difficulty in breathing
- Vomiting with blood
- Painful urination with back pain
- Severe headache, if associated with a fever and possibly with a rash
- Severe headache that develops very suddenly
- Difficulty in swallowing saliva
- Central, crushing chest pain in adult
- Nosebleed for more than 30 minutes, despite first-aid measures
- An object, such as a bead, up the nose of a child (but not if in the ear)
- Bee sting near or in the mouth
- Swallowed detergents or poisons
- Chemicals in the eye

# Homeopathy

Nearly 200 years ago Samuel Hahnemann found that a medicine that causes symptoms in a healthy person could, in small doses, help cure those same symptoms in a sick person. It is therefore important to match your symptoms with those associated with the remedy. Whatever makes the pain better or worse offers a useful pointer to individualize the symptom picture and thus select the correct remedy.

There are too many symptoms associated with each remedy to list them in full throughout the book, but a few important ones are given under each ailment as guides. Try the remedy that appears to match your symptoms. If the symptoms change, consult the remedy pictures again. It is always best to consult a qualified homeopath, who can pre-scribe a remedy based on you as an individual.

Homeopathic remedies are prepared by serial dilutions of a solution of the remedy in alcohol, or are mixed with lactose until they become soluble. Two scales are commonly used: the decimal (x) scale and the centesimal (c) scale, used throughout this book. Remedies are usually sold in 6c or 30c potency. The higher the dilution, the greater its strength. The choice of preparation is a personal one – powders can be dissolved in water or tablets crushed. A small amount of the liquid or crushed tablet comprises one dose. Remedies can also be bought as creams or solutions to put on the skin.

**BELOW** Homeopathic remedies are usually stored in dark glass bottles.

All remedies should be stored in a cool, dry place, away from strong-smelling substances. Tablets should never be handled – instead, tip one onto the lid of the bottle, then straight into your mouth. Remedies should be sucked, not swallowed. Have nothing strong-tasting in your mouth before taking the remedy, and nothing to eat or drink for 10 minutes before or after.

# Most useful homeopathic remedies

**ARGENTUM NITRICUM** For anxiety, chronic fatigue syndrome, depression, gastritis, IBS, laryngitis.

**ARSENICUM ALBUM** For diarrhoea and vomiting, food poisoning, gastritis, peptic ulcers, eczema, psoriasis, hay fever, asthma.

**BELLADONNA** For earache, fever, tonsillitis, arthritis, German measles, scarlet fever.

**BRYONIA** For gastritis, indigestion, chest infections, sciatica, headache.

**CHAMOMILLA** For earache, teething, colic, cough, painful periods, toothache.

**GELSEMIUM** For fear of dentist/driving test, anxiety symptoms generally, flu, diarrhoea, chronic fatigue syndrome.

**HEPAR SULPHURIS** For abscesses, acne, sore throat, coughs and bronchitis, earache.

**IGNATIA** For grief, cough, depression, headache.

**IPECACUANHA** For asthma, cough, nausea in pregnancy.

**LACHESIS** For asthma, flushes and menopausal problems, heavy periods, sore throats.

**LYCOPODIUM** For bowel problems, bloating, IBS, heartburn, migraine, urinary infection, premature baldness.

**MERCURIUS** For mouth ulcers, colds, sore throat, colitis, ear infections, ulcerative colitis.

**NATRUM MURIATICUM** For mouth ulcers, cold sores, asthma, eczema, psoriasis, IBS, headaches, PMS.

**NUX VOMICA** For stress, overwork, fatigue, insomnia, hay fever, asthma, colic, IBS, headaches, peptic ulcers.

**PHOSPHORUS** For peptic ulcers, gastritis, colitis, coughs and bronchitis, nosebleeds.

**PULSATILLA** For pregnancy sickness, breech presentations, cystitis, postnatal depression, period problems, hay fever, conjunctivitis, recurrent ear infections, IBS, bedwetting.

**RHUS TOXICODENDRON** For chickenpox, shingles, arthritis, rheumatism, eczema, sprains.

**SEPIA** For depression, fatigue, cystitis, PMS, back pain, nausea in pregnancy, warts, ringworm.

**STAPHYSAGRIA** For depression, cystitis related to intercourse, PMS, psoriasis (particularly after grief), warts, pain in surgical wounds.

**SULPHUR** For abscesses, acne, eczema, asthma, dandruff, menopausal flushes, migraine, arthritis, tonsillitis.

# Aromatherapy

LAVENDER

## ESSENTIAL OILS

Essential oils are extracted from the leaves, fruit, flowers, bark, roots and wood of plants and trees and are absorbed by the body during aromatherapy, either through inhalation or the pores of the skin.

## Caution

*Never ingest essential oils or apply them neat to the skin (unless specifically suggested in the text), as they can cause irritation.*

## BASE / CARRIER OILS

For direct skin application, mix essential oils with a base, or carrier, oil. This enables them to penetrate the skin without causing irritation or burning. Any of the light vegetable-based oils that you put in your mouth you can put on your skin.

## MASSAGE OILS

To make a massage oil, add 2 drops of essential oil to 5ml/1tsp of carrier oil, or to 5ml/1tsp of aqueous cream or lotion. For a child, add 1 drop of essential oil to 10ml/2tsp of carrier oil or cream.

## STEAM INHALATIONS

Add 4–6 drops of essential oil to a bowl of hot water. Bend over the bowl, cover your head with a towel and inhale the steam. This treatment is not suitable for asthmatics or small children. Alternatively, put 1–2 drops of oil on a handkerchief or pillow; or run the hot tap into the bath and sit in the steamy bathroom with a child.

## COMPRESSES

Add 4–6 drops of essential oil to a bowl of warm water and mix well. Soak the compress, then squeeze out the excess water (but do not wring). Apply to the affected area. If possible, wrap in clingfilm followed by a warm towel. Keep covered for at least 2 hours (preferably overnight).

## BATHING WITH OILS

Run the bath, then add 4–6 drops of oil for adults and 1–2 drops for children (or mix with a carrier oil or milk first). Agitate the water, then soak for at least 20 minutes. Follow the same process for foot, hand and sitz baths.

## VAPORIZERS

Never allow your burner to run dry or leave it unattended, as some essential oils are highly flammable. Put 1–2 drops of oil into the vaporizer and heat for 15–20 minutes. Then turn the vaporizer off, or blow out the candle. The effects will last for 4–6 hours. Alternatively, soak a piece of cottonwool in 1–2 drops of oil and place behind a warm radiator.

## SPRAYS

Put 10–15 drops of essential oil into 1l/1¾ pt of water, then spray lightly over the area. This is very useful if the area is too painful to be touched.

# Most useful aromatherapeutic oils

**BASIL** Mind-clearing and focusing – useful to help studying, or for switching off at the end of a busy day; clearing to the sinus.

**CLOVE** Good for toothache; in a burner at festive occasions, used with orange, pine and/or cinnamon.

**EUCALYPTUS** Beneficial for cold, flu and sinus problems; good as a massage medium or in the bath for muscular aches and pains.

**FRANKINCENSE** Soothing to the emotions; slows and deepens the breathing; good for asthmatics in a vaporizer or on a handkerchief.

**GERANIUM** For all women's problems, especially those to do with hormonal imbalance (PMS and the menopause).

**GINGER** Warming to the muscles; beneficial for digestive disorders; good for all nausea.

**JASMINE** Eases labour pains; useful for postnatal blues.

**JUNIPER** Detoxifying, both mentally and physically.

**LAVENDER** Calming, soothing, relaxing, de-stressing; useful for burns and insomnia.

**LEMON** Good for treating both warts and verrucae.

**LEMON GRASS** Builds the body's resistance to fatigue; good in a foot bath for tired, restless legs; an effective insect repellent.

**MANDARIN** Safe and gentle, relaxing for everyone; a valuable general oil.

**NEROLI** The best oil for stress-related problems.

**ORANGE** A sunny, cheering oil – uplifting and joyful.

**PETITGRAIN** Good for stress conditions, where neroli is indicated but is unaffordable.

**ROMAN CAMOMILE** I drop in a bath soothes a fractious child at bedtime; beneficial for skin irritations; good in a tea for digestive disorders.

**ROSE** The ultimate feminine oil for menstrual disruption; beneficial for emotional stress and grief.

**SANDALWOOD** Soothing to the skin and the emotions; good for massaging (mixed with a carrier oil or lotion) in the throat area.

**TEA TREE** Antiviral, antifungal and antibacterial; good for warts, verrucae, athlete's foot and boosting the immune system.

**YLANG YLANG** Antidepressant – a heady oil, purportedly an aphrodisiac.

# Most useful healing foods

CARROT

**APPLES** Good for the heart; protective against pollution; lower cholesterol; good for food poisoning and for gastroenteritis; antibacterial and antiviral; their fibre helps digestion.

APPLE

**ARTICHOKES (GLOBE)** Good for liver complaints, biliousness, hepatitis and gallstones; lower cholesterol; relieve fluid retention; excellent for rheumatism, arthritis and gout.

**AVOCADOS** Ideal convalescing food; good for stress and sexual problems; excellent for skin conditions; powerfully antioxidant and protective against heart disease and cancers; contain a valuable antibacterial and antifungal chemical.

**BANANAS** Excellent for the physically active and for anyone taking diuretics; good for PMS; very healing for the whole digestive tract; good for both constipation and diarrhoea.

AVOCADO

BANANA

**CABBAGE** The medicine of the poor – use cabbage juice for peptic ulcers; cabbage leaves as compresses for painful joints; cabbage soup for chest infections; the dark green leaves for anaemia. Cabbage and all its relatives are powerful protectors against a whole range of cancers.

**CARROTS** Good for the eyes; useful puréed to treat infant diarrhoea; excellent for liver problems; great for healthy skin; protective against heart disease and lung cancer.

**GARLIC** The king of healing plants – antibacterial, antifungal, and good for everything from bronchitis to athlete's foot; protective against food poisoning; lowers cholesterol and blood pressure; improves circulation.

**KIWI FRUIT** Good for blood pressure, digestive problems, chronic fatigue and heart problems.

**LEEKS** Beneficial for all breathing problems; cleansing and diuretic; excellent for gout, arthritis and for rheumatism.

**LEMONS, ORANGES AND GRAPEFRUITS** Valuable in the treatment of coughs, colds and flu; in strengthening natural immunity.

**NUTS** The healing plants and trees of tomorrow and densely full of nutrients – minerals like selenium, zinc, iron, lots of protein, healthy oils and the B vitamins. Fresh, unsalted nuts should form a daily part of everyone's diet.

**OATS** Contain a cornucopia of nutrients; the best anti-constipation food; also lower cholesterol; help control blood pressure; have a calming effect on the mind and a healing effect on the stomach.

**OLIVE OIL (EXTRA-VIRGIN)** A remarkable food/medicine – lowers cholesterol; protects against cell damage; increases the level of the healthy blood fats that scavenge bad fats from the arteries; good for liver and gall-bladder problems; protective against arthritis, senility and even against some cancers.

**ONIONS** From the same family as leeks and garlic; important in the treatment of all chest infections; should be eaten by anyone who has high blood pressure, raised cholesterol or heart disease; an excellent food for anaemia, asthma, urinary infections – and even for helping with hangovers.

**PINEAPPLES** Like the other tropical fruits, such as mangoes and pawpaws, much underrated for its health benefits; ideal for sore throats, joint diseases, digestive problems and all muscular injuries.

**PULSES (DRIED PEAS, BEANS AND LENTILS)** Protective against heart disease and cancers (especially of the bowel); excellent for constipation, fatigue, chronic fatigue syndrome and diabetes.

**RICE** Perfect food for convalescents, those with digestive problems, stress and exhaustion. Brown rice is also important in the treatment of circulatory disorders. Plain boiled rice lowers cholesterol and is ideal as a treatment for diarrhoea.

**WATERCRESS** A great protector against cancer; powerfully antibiotic, without killing off the natural bacteria; helps with urinary infections; a good stimulant of the thyroid gland.

**WHEAT** Highly protective against bowel disease, high blood pressure, constipation and stress-related illnesses. Sprouted wheat seeds help in the fight against cancer. Bread can also be used as a hot poultice for boils, abscesses and splinters.

**YOGURT (LIVE)** Protective against stomach infections, food poisoning and constipation; boosts the immune system and should be eaten by those with viral or bacterial illnesses; protective against fungal infections like thrush.

PEANUTS

PINEAPPLE

# Food combining:
## the Hay diet

There are many misconceptions surrounding the food combining, or Hay, diet. It is not the panacea for all ills, but it can be very beneficial for people with digestive complaints. Try it for a couple of weeks and see if it suits you – a bonus is that anyone who is overweight will certainly lose a few pounds.

The only rule that really matters is not combining starch foods and protein foods in the same meal. For example: no fish (protein) and chips (starch); no meat (protein) and potatoes (starch). Allow 3 hours between meals and if you want to snack, choose from the neutral list, which can be eaten with either starch or protein.

| PROTEIN FOODS | STARCH FOODS |
|---|---|
| meat | potatoes and yams |
| poultry | sweetcorn |
| game | bread and flour |
| fish and shellfish | oats, wheat and barley |
| eggs | rice |
| fruit (except those listed in the starch group) | millet and rye |
| peanuts | buckwheat |
| soya beans | pasta |
| tofu | very sweet fruit, such as ripe pears |
| milk | bananas |
| yogurt | papaya and mangoes |
| all cheese (except cream cheese and ricotta) | sweet grapes |
| wine and cider | beer |

| NEUTRAL FOODS | |
|---|---|
| all vegetables (except those listed in the starch group) | beans and chickpeas (but not soya beans) |
| all nuts (except peanuts) | all seeds and sprouted seeds |
| butter and cream | herbs and spices |
| cream cheese and ricotta | raisins and sultanas |
| egg yolk | honey and maple syrup |
| olive, sesame and sunflower oils | (yogurt and milk have a very low protein |
| lentils and split peas | content, so they can be used in tiny |
| | amounts with starch foods) |

# The exclusion diet

sIf you have a 'food intolerance', try this exclusion diet for a couple of weeks. If it does not help, seek professional help. If it does help, start adding foods back one at a time to see which, if any, causes your symptoms. Exclude any culprit foods for a few months, then try them again, but any long-term removal of major food groups should only be done under professional guidance. During the first 2 weeks of the diet follow this chart to see which foods you may, and may not, eat.

| FOOD | NOT ALLOWED | ALLOWED |
|------|-------------|---------|
| MEAT | preserved meats, bacon, sausages, all processed meat products | all other meats |
| FISH | smoked fish, shellfish | white fish |
| VEGETABLES | potatoes, onions, sweetcorn, aubergines, sweet peppers, chillies, tomatoes | all other vegetables, salads, pulses, swedes, parsnips |
| FRUIT | citrus fruit (e.g. oranges, grapefruit) | all other fruit (e.g. apples, bananas, pears) |
| CEREALS | wheat, oats, barley, rye, corn | rice, ground rice, rice flakes, rice flour, sago, rice breakfast cereals, tapioca, millet, buckwheat, rice cakes |
| COOKING OILS | corn oil, vegetable oil | sunflower oil, soya oil, safflower oil, olive oil |
| DAIRY PRODUCTS | cow's milk, butter, most margarines, cow's milk yogurt and cheese, eggs | goat, sheep and soya milk and products made from them, dairy and trans fat-free margarines |
| BEVERAGES | tea, coffee (beans, instant and decaffeinated), fruit squashes, orange juice, grapefruit juice, alcohol and tap water | herbal teas (e.g. camomile), fresh fruit juices (e.g. apple, pineapple), pure tomato juice (without additives), mineral, distilled or de-ionized water |
| MISCELLANEOUS | chocolates, yeast, yeast extracts, artificial preservatives, colourings and flavourings, monosodium glutamate, all artificial sweeteners | carob, sea salt, herbs, spices and small amounts of sugar or honey |

After 2 weeks introduce other foods in this order: tap water, potatoes, cow's milk, yeast, tea, rye, butter, onions, eggs, porridge oats, coffee, chocolate, barley, citrus fruit, corn, cow's cheese, white wine, shellfish, natural cow's milk yogurt, vinegar, wheat and nuts.

# Home medicine chest

Every medicine chest needs the normal range of bandages, plasters, safety pins, antiseptic, tweezers and scissors, together with a supply of proprietary painkillers, anti-diarrhoeals, and so on.

However, the home medicine chest recommended here includes many other natural ingredients, as powerful aids to the safe and effective treatment of most minor ailments.

## ✚ CONVENTIONAL REMEDIES

- Calamine lotion
- Chlorpheniramine maleate
- Clotrimazole cream
- Hydrocortisone 1% cream
- Ibuprofen
- Oral rehydration powder sachets (for reconstitution in case of diarrhoea)
- Paracetamol

## 🍃 HERBAL REMEDIES

- A potted *Aloe vera* plant to grow on a sunny windowsill
- Arnica cream
- Camomile flowers – loose or in teabags
- Chickweed cream
- Echinacea tablets
- Lavender oil
- Marigold cream
- Meadowsweet tincture
- Myrrh tincture
- Slippery-elm tablets
- Tea-tree oil
- Distilled witch hazel (or alternatively witch-hazel tincture)

## ✿ HOMEOPATHIC REMEDIES

All at 6c potency and 30c potency.

- Aconite
- Arnica
- Apis
- Belladonna
- Bellis perennis
- Cantharis
- Hypercal ointment
- Hypericum
- Ledum
- Rhus toxicodendrum
- Silicea
- Symphytum
- Urtica urens

## 💧 AROMATHERAPY OILS

It is not worth storing large quantities of essential oils, as they have a shelf-life of only 1–2 years, so unless you are going to use them regularly, do not keep a large stock of them in your medicine chest. Buy oils that have a multitude of uses for you and your family, such as the ones listed below, or oils to help specific ailments, as suggested throughout the book.

- Eucalyptus
- Lavender
- Tea tree

## KITCHEN REMEDIES

- Cider vinegar
- Cinnamon
- Cloves
- Epsom salts
- Garlic (fresh)
- Ginger root
- Horseradish
- Mustard powder
- Organic honey
- Sage (either a plant or dried)
- Sodium bicarbonate
- Teabags

**LEFT** Treat minor ailments from your home medicine chest.

# Useful addresses

## AROMATHERAPY
### Europe
ACADEMY OF AROMATHERAPY
AND MASSAGE
50 Cow Wynd
Falkirk
Stirlingshire FK1 1PU
Great Britain
Tel: 44 1324 612658

INTERNATIONAL FEDERATION
OF AROMATHERAPISTS
Stamford House
2–4 Chiswick High Road
London W4 1TH
Great Britain
Tel: 44 208 742 2605
Fax: 44 208 742 2606

INTERNATIONAL SOCIETY
OF PROFESSIONAL
AROMATHERAPISTS
ISPA House
82 Ashby Road
Hinckley
Leics OE10 1SN
Great Britain
Tel: 44 1455 637987
Fax: 44 1455 890956

TISSERAND INSTITUTE
65 Church Road
Hove
East Sussex BN3 2BD
Great Britain
Tel: 44 1273 206640
Fax: 44 1273 329811

### North America
AMERICAN ALLIANCE
OF AROMATHERAPY
PO Box 750428
Petaluma
California 94975-0428
USA
Tel: 1 707 778 6762
Fax: 1 707 769 0868

AMERICAN AROMATHERAPY
ASSOCIATION
PO Box 3679
South Pasadena
California 91031
USA
Tel: 1 818 457 1742

NATIONAL ASSOCIATION OF
HOLISTIC AROMATHERAPY
PO Box 17622
Boulder
Colorado 80308-0622
USA
Tel: 1 303 258 3791

## CONVENTIONAL MEDICINE
### Australasia
SKIN AND PSORIASIS
FOUNDATION
OF VICTORIA
PO Box 228
Collins Street
PO 3000
Melbourne 671962
Victoria
Australia

### Europe
ARTHRITIS AND RHEUMATISM
COUNCIL FOR RESEARCH
Copeman House
St Mary's Court
St Mary's Gate
Chesterfield S41 7TD
Great Britain
Tel: 44 1246 558033

BRITISH MIGRAINE ASSOCIATION
178a High Road
Byfleet
West Byfleet
Surrey KT14 7ED
Great Britain
Tel: 44 1932 352468

ENURESIS RESOURCE AND
INFORMATION CENTRE
65 St Michael's Hill
Bristol BS2 8DZ
Great Britain
Tel: 44 117 9264920

HAIRLINE INTERNATIONAL: THE
ALOPECIA PATIENTS' SOCIETY
Lyon's Court
1668 High Street
Knowle
West Midlands B93 0LY
Great Britain
Tel: 44 1564 775281

HERPES ASSOCIATION
41 North Road
London N7 9DP
Great Britain
Tel: 44 207 607 9661
(Helpline: 44 207 609 9061)

MEDIC ALERT FOUNDATION
12 Bridge Wharf
156 Caledonian Road
London N1 9UU
Great Britain
Tel: 44 207 833 3034

NATIONAL ASTHMA CAMPAIGN
Providence House
Providence Place
London N1 0NT
Great Britain
Tel: 44 207 226 2260

NATIONAL BACK PAIN ASSOCIATION
16 Elmtree Road
Teddington
Middlesex TW11 8ST
Great Britain
Tel: 44 208 977 5474

NATIONAL ECZEMA SOCIETY
4 Tavistock Place
London WC1H 9RA
Great Britain
Tel: 44 207 388 4097

NATIONAL OSTEOPOROSIS SOCIETY
PO Box 10
Radstock
Bath BA3 3YB
Great Britain
Tel: 44 1761 432472

PATIENTS' ASSOCIATION
PO Box 935
Harrow
Middlesex HA1 3YJ
Great Britain
Helpline: 44 208 423 8999

PSORIASIS ASSOCIATION
7 Milton Street
Northampton NN2 7JG
Great Britain
Tel: 44 1604 711129

SEASONAL AFFECTIVE DISORDER
ASSOCIATION
PO Box 989
London SW7 2PZ
Great Britain
Tel: 44 208 969 7028

SENSE NATIONAL DEAFBLIND
AND RUBELLA ASSOCIATION
11–13 Clifton Terrace
Finsbury Park
London N4 3SR
Great Britain
Tel: 44 207 272 7774

SOCIETY OF CHIROPODISTS
53 Welbeck Street
London W1M 7HE
Great Britain
Tel: 44 207 486 3381

WOMEN'S HEALTH CONCERN
83 Earls Court Road
London W8 6EF
Great Britain
Tel: 44 207 938 3932

### North America
NATIONAL PSORIASIS FOUNDATION
Suite 200
6415 South West Canyon Court
Portland, Oregon 97221
USA
Tel: 1 503 297 1545

## HERBALISM
### Australasia
NATIONAL HERBALISTS
ASSOCIATION OF AUSTRALIA
Suite 305, BST House
3 Smail Street
Broadway
New South Wales 2007
Australia
Tel: 61 2 211 6437
Fax: 61 2 211 6452

### Europe
BRITISH HERBAL MEDICINE
ASSOCIATION
1 Wickham Road
Boscombe
Bournemouth
Dorset BH7 6JX
Great Britain
Tel: 44 1202 433691

THE HERB SOCIETY
Deddington Hill Farm
Warmington
Banbury
Oxon OX17 1XB
Great Britain
Tel: 44 1295 692900

NATIONAL INSTITUTE OF
MEDICAL HERBALISTS
56 Longbrook Street
Exeter
Devon EX4 6AH
Great Britain
Tel: 44 1392 426022

SCHOOL OF HERBAL
MEDICINE/PHYTOTHERAPY
Bucksteep Manor
Bodle Street Green
Near Hailsham
Sussex BN27 4RJ
Great Britain
Tel: 44 1323 834 800
Fax: 44 1323 834 801

### North America
AMERICAN BOTANICAL COUNCIL
PO Box 201660
Austin
Texas 78720-1660
USA
Tel: 1 512 331 1924

AMERICAN HERBALISTS GUILD
PO Box 1683
Soquel
California 95073
USA

## HOMEOPATHY
### Australasia
AUSTRALIAN HOMEOPATHIC
ASSOCIATION
11 Landsborough Terrace
Toowong 4006
Australia
Tel/Fax: 61 7 3371 7245
e-mail: vikiwill@powerup.com.au

AUSTRALIAN INSTITUTE
OF HOMEOPATHY
21 Bulah Heights
Berdwra Heights
New South Wales 2082
Australia

NEW ZEALAND INSTITUTE OF
CLASSICAL HOMEOPATHY
PO Box 7232
Wellesley Street
Auckland
New Zealand
e-mail: jwinston@actrix.gen.nz

### Europe
BRITISH HOMOEOPATHIC
ASSOCIATION
27A Devonshire Street
London W1N 1RJ
Great Britain
Tel: 44 207 935 2163

CENTRE D'ETUDES
Homéopathiques de France
228 Boulevard Raspail
75014 Paris
France
Tel: 33 143 207896

FACULTY OF HOMEOPATHY
Hahnemann House
2 Powis Place
London WC1N 3HT
Great Britain
Tel: 44 207 837 9469

SOCIÉTÉ MÉDICAL DE
BIOTHÉRAPIE
62 rue Beaubourg
75003 Paris
France
Tel: 33 143 346000

SOCIETY OF HOMOEOPATHS
2 Artisan Road
Northampton NN1 4HU
Great Britain
Tel: 44 1604 21400
Fax: 44 1604 22622

### North America
HOMEOPATHIC ASSOCIATION
OF NATUROPATHIC
PHYSICIANS (HANP)
PO Box 69565
Portland
Oregon 97201
USA
Tel: 1 503 795 0579

NATIONAL CENTER FOR
HOMEOPATHY
801 North Fairfax Street
Suite 306
Alexandria
Virginia 22314
USA
Tel: 1 703 548 7790
Fax: 1 703 548 7792
e-mail: nch@igc.org

NORTH AMERICAN SOCIETY OF
HOMEOPATHS (NASH)
2024 S. Dearborn Street
Seattle
Washington 98144-2912
USA
Tel: 1 206 720 7000
Fax: 1 206 329 5684
e-mail: NashInfo@aol.com
Website: www.homeopathy.org

## NUTRITION
### Europe
THE BRITISH NATUROPATHIC
ASSOCIATION
Frazer House
6 Netherhall Gardens
London NW3 5RR
Great Britain
Tel: 44 207 435 7830

EATING DISORDERS ASSOCIATION
Sackville Place
44 Magdalen Street
Norwich NR3 1JU
Great Britain
Helpline: 44 1603 621414
Fax: 44 1603 664915
Website: www.gurney.org.uk/eda/

VEGETARIAN SOCIETY
Parkdale
Dunham Road
Altrincham
Cheshire WA14 4QG
Great Britain
Tel: 44 161 928 4QG
Fax: 44 161 926 9182

### North America
AMERICAN ASSOCIATION OF
NUTRITION CONSULTANTS
1641 East Sunset Road,
Apt B-117
Las Vegas
Nevada 89119
USA
Tel: 1 709 361 1132

AMERICAN DIETETICS
ASSOCIATION
216 West Jackson Boulevard
Apt 800
Chicago
Illinois 60606-6995
USA
Tel: 1 800 877 1600

EATING DISORDERS AWARENESS
AND PREVENTION
603 Steward Street
Suite 8013
Seattle
Washington 98101
USA
Tel: 1 206 382 3587

NORTH AMERICAN VEGETARIAN
SOCIETY
PO Box 72
Dolgeville
New York NY 13329
USA
Tel: 1 518 568 7970

# Index

# Contributors

**NAOMI CRAFT,** Bsc, MBBS, MRCGP, qualified in 1988 and is now a general practitioner in London. A regular contributor to self-help books, she has also written for magazines and newspapers and has appeared on television and radio. In 1996 she received an award for excellence from the Medical Journalists' Association.

**JOSIE DRAKE,** ITEC, PhysETh, AIPTI, LTPhys, is a highly qualified therapist who specializes in teaching massage, aromatherapy, diet nutrition and stress management. She has also worked at Stoke Mandeville Hospital and was acclaimed the 1997 National Health and Beauty's Community Therapist of the Year.

**DR FIONA DRY,** MBBS, MRCGP, DSMSA, MFHom is a general practitioner and homeopath based in Leighton Buzzard, Bedfordshire. She also works as a sports physician for the Badminton Association of England, with their élite athletes.

**PENELOPE ODY** is a member of the National Institute of Medical Herbalists and a Fellow of the Herb Society, and ran her own herbal practice in Buckinghamshire for 12 years. She has written books on herbal medicine and home remedies, and lectures widely on these themes.

**C. NORMAN SHEALY,** MD, PhD, is founding President of the American Holistic Medical Association and of the Shealy Center, America's foremost alternative-medicine clinic.

**MICHAEL VAN STRATEN** is a registered naturopath, osteopath and acupuncturist and a former governor of the British College of Naturopathy and Osteopathy. The author of many books on nutrition and natural health, he is also a health journalist writing for newspapers and magazines, and a prolific radio and TV broadcaster. He also runs his own naturopathy practices in London and Buckinghamshire.